SYMPOSIA OF THE SECTION ON MICROBIOLOGY
THE NEW YORK ACADEMY OF MEDICINE

Number 6
THE EFFECT OF ACTH AND CORTISONE UPON INFECTION AND RESISTANCE

THE EFFECT OF ACTH AND CORTISONE UPON INFECTION AND RESISTANCE

EDITED BY

Gregory Shwartzman, M.D.

SYMPOSIUM HELD AT THE
NEW YORK ACADEMY OF MEDICINE
MARCH 27 and 28, 1952

1953   New York
COLUMBIA UNIVERSITY PRESS

COPYRIGHT 1953 NEW YORK
COLUMBIA UNIVERSITY PRESS

PUBLISHED IN GREAT BRITAIN,
CANADA, INDIA, AND PAKISTAN
BY GEOFFREY CUMBERLEGE,
OXFORD UNIVERSITY PRESS,
LONDON, TORONTO, BOMBAY, AND KARACHI

The Selman A. Waksman Foundation has made possible the publication of this symposium through a generous grant to meet part of the cost

MANUFACTURED IN THE UNITED STATES OF AMERICA

SECTION ON MICROBIOLOGY
THE NEW YORK ACADEMY OF MEDICINE

Officers
COLIN M. MACLEOD, *Chairman*
JOHN G. KIDD, *Secretary*

Advisory Board
THOMAS P. MAGILL
WALSH MCDERMOTT
RALPH S. MUCKENFUSS
BEATRICE CARRIER SEEGAL
GREGORY SHWARTZMAN

Organizing Committee for Symposium Number 6
GREGORY SHWARTZMAN, *Chairman*
JOHN G. KIDD
ROBERT F. LOEB

Foreword

ON MAY 1, 1947, the Fellowship of The New York Academy of Medicine approved the organization of the Section on Microbiology, thus establishing the first section of the Academy devoted to basic medical sciences.

Ample opportunities are already available for presentation and publication of scientific papers. However, with increasing diversity, complexity, and specialization, there is evident a need for opportunity to digest and correlate the rapidly accumulating body of new knowledge The main objectives of the new Section are to provide a forum for the exchange of information amongst the workers engaged in basic and clinical sciences.

Accordingly, the scope of interest of the Section on Microbiology is broadly defined as embodying the following: (1) bacteriology, mycology, and parasitology; (2) viruses and rickettsiae; (3) maladies of unknown or uncertain etiology, possibly of infectious origin; (4) immunology; (5) chemotherapy; (6) pathology relative to microbiology; and (7) methods of study adopted from related sciences as applied to microbiology. The programs of meetings of the Section are arranged to deal with single topics in their various aspects. In addition to regular monthly evening meetings, several symposia are organized yearly, each consisting of consecutive afternoon and evening sessions. The participants present extensive reviews in their particular fields of endeavor, thus bringing correlated and authoritative scientific data and concepts to the attention of the microbiologists and allied laboratory and clinical investigators. Symposia are soon forgotten if they are not published, but their benefits may be retained by prompt publication. Important service is rendered by the Columbia University Press, which has undertaken the publication of this series under the auspices of the New York Academy of Medicine and the editorship of the respective chairmen of the symposia.

GREGORY SHWARTZMAN

New York, N.Y.
April, 1953

Contents

1. INTRODUCTION 3
   Gregory Shwartzman, *Mount Sinai Hospital*

2. SOME GENERAL CONSIDERATIONS CONCERNING THE ROLE OF THE ADRENAL CORTEX IN INTERMEDIARY METABOLISM 6
   Frank L. Engel, *Duke University*

3. THE INFLUENCE OF ADRENALECTOMY AND CORTISONE TREATMENT ON CERTAIN ENZYMATIC REACTIONS IN THE RAT 17
   W. W. Umbreit, *The Merck Institute for Therapeutic Research*

4. THE EFFECT OF CORTICOSTEROIDS UPON LYMPHOID TISSUE 25
   William E. Ehrich and Joseph Seifter, *University of Pennsylvania, Philadelphia General Hospital, and Wyeth Institute of Applied Biochemistry*

5. THE EFFECT OF CORTISONE UPON REPAIR PROCESSES IN DENSE AND LOOSE CONNECTIVE TISSUE 46
   Charles Ragan, Raffael Lattes, J. W. Blunt, Jr., de Guise Vaillancourt, Ralph A. Jessar, and Wallace Epstein, *College of Physicians and Surgeons, Columbia University, and Presbyterian Hospital*

6. ADRENAL HORMONES AND THE DEVELOPMENT OF ANTIBODY AND HYPERSENSITIVITY 56
   Edward E. Fischel, *College of Physicians and Surgeons, Columbia University, and Presbyterian Hospital*

7. DEPRESSION BY CORTISONE OF INHERITED AND ACQUIRED RESISTANCE TO INFECTION AND TO TUMOR GRAFTING 72
   Herbert C. Stoerk, *The Merck Institute for Therapeutic Research*

8. CONSTITUTIONAL FACTORS IN RESISTANCE TO INFECTION; THE EFFECT OF CORTISONE ON THE PATHOGENESIS OF TUBERCULOSIS   84
Max B. Lurie, Peter Zappasodi, Arthur M. Dannenberg, Jr., and Eugenia Cardona-Lynch, *The Henry Phipps Institute, University of Pennsylvania*

9. STUDIES ON THE MECHANISM OF ACTION OF CORTISONE IN EXPERIMENTAL SYPHILIS   100
Thomas B. Turner and David H. Hollander, *The Johns Hopkins University School of Hygiene and Public Health*

10. THE EFFECT OF CORTISONE IN ACTIVATING LATENT TRYPANOSOMIASIS IN RHESUS MONKEYS   122
Abner Wolf, Elvin A. Kabat, Ada E. Bezer, and James R. C. Fonseca, *College of Physicians and Surgeons, Columbia University, and Presbyterian Hospital*

11. THE EFFECT OF ACTH AND CORTISONE UPON ALLERGIC DISEASES   140
A. McGehee Harvey, Lawrence E. Shulman, and Edith H. Schoenrich, *The Johns Hopkins University School of Medicine*

12. THE EFFECTS OF CORTISONE ON BACTERIAL INFECTION AND INTOXICATION   147
Lewis Thomas, *University of Minnesota Medical School*

13. OBSERVATIONS ON ADRENAL CORTICAL HORMONES IN PNEUMOCOCCAL AND INFLUENZA VIRAL INFECTIONS AND IN MALARIA   161
Edward H. Kass, *National Research Council*, Quentin M. Geiman, and Maxwell Finland

14. ALTERATION OF EXPERIMENTAL POLIOMYELITIS BY MEANS OF CORTISONE WITH REFERENCE TO OTHER VIRUSES   176
Gregory Shwartzman and Stanley M. Aronson, *Mount Sinai Hospital*

THE EFFECT OF ACTH AND CORTISONE
UPON INFECTION AND RESISTANCE

Chapter 1

INTRODUCTION

BY GREGORY SHWARTZMAN

IN ORDER TO GRASP the significance of the impact which may be produced in the near future by the information to be presented at this symposium it may be well to recall the periodical shifts in interest which succeeded one another during the past fifty years in the sciences dealing with infection and resistance. It was only natural for investigators to be impressed by discoveries of specific causes of diseases and specific reactions of the body to these diseases. This was an era best defined as the era of "specificity." Thus, the main emphasis was laid upon the invading agent, its behavior and characteristics, and the response of the body to the invader expressing itself in specific antibodies. As fruitful as this trend was, impasses began to appear. Consequently, many departures from previous thinking resulted from a large body of evidence concerned with variations in predisposition and resistance to disease which could not be explained on the basis of specific immunity, namely: refractoriness of certain animal species to highly infectious agents; variations in susceptibility to disease within the same animal species which could not be accounted for by the presence or absence of antibodies; variations contingent upon genetic selections, seasonal variations, selective affinities for various tissues and organs, variations in age susceptibility, and so forth.

When considered together, these facts indicate the existence of important factors unrelated to specific immunity which may determine the predisposition or resistance of the host. In other words, the time has come to shift our interest from the causative agent to the host.

Although the possible role of hormones in predisposition and resistance to disease has been long suspected, previous studies, especially in reference to adrenocortical function, were at best equivocal, mainly because adrenocortical extracts of low and variable potency and representing mixtures of various hormones were used. The effect of adrenalectomy on resistance to infection, although a subject of prolonged investigation, failed to give clear-cut information beyond the fact that the absence of the adrenal cortex renders the host extremely susceptible to a variety of toxic and infectious agents, while administration of adrenocortical extracts may restore the normal resistance of the adrenalectomized animal.

However, the attempts in this direction have gained a considerable impetus from the isolation and physiological identification of adrenocortical and adrenocorticotrophic hormones. Shortly after the introduction of the hormones for clinical use, the investigators were so impressed with the beneficial therapeutic effect of the hormones on certain diseases that the initial experimental studies were primarily designed to test their curative value in bacterial and viral diseases. It was soon found that the hormones exerted no protective effect. By reversing the conditions of the experiments some investigators were able to demonstrate the opposite effect, the enhancement of infections.

Although the investigations about to be reported at this symposium will deal primarily with the effect of ACTH and cortisone upon infection and resistance, the Organizing Committee deemed it important to devote a portion of the time to general considerations of the action of the hormones, namely, their effect upon metabolic functions and structural elements of the organism, with the hope that the knowledge of these basic facts will aid us in the understanding of the mechanism of the effect of the hormones upon infection and resistance. The structural changes produced by the hormones are likely to attract our attention first. Although very interesting and important, they have to be viewed as a morphological expression of the profound physiological role which the hormones play in many metabolic functions. There may be, indeed, different phases of these functions concerned with the relationship of the host to various viral and bacterial invaders.

It will be demonstrated at this symposium that in some infections the effects of ACTH and cortisone are similar, while in others, differences exist between the action of the two hormones. In the evaluation of the results it may be well to remember the basic differences between the physiological action of these hormones.

Under normal conditions adrenocortical function represents a delicately balanced hormonal system capable of elaborating a variety of adrenocortical hormones. ACTH stimulates the adrenal cortex as a whole, thus apparently eliciting the production of a number of hormones in addition to cortisone or compound F. In sharp contrast, the

INTRODUCTION 5

administration of cortisone results in a depression of the function of the adrenal cortex, presumably depriving the body of adrenocortical hormones other than cortisone. The differences beween the effects of ACTH and cortisone may thus be due to the ability of some adrenocortical hormones to oppose the action of cortisone. This is merely a working hypothesis.

At this stage we can do no more than to branch out over a single plane and hope to arrive slowly through differentiation at the understanding of this new field. Further progress may be facilitated if we avoid generalizations. But I am sure you will all agree that we are about to enter a new and fascinating field of studies on host-parasite relationships.

Chapter 2

SOME GENERAL CONSIDERATIONS CONCERNING THE ROLE OF THE ADRENAL CORTEX IN INTERMEDIARY METABOLISM

By Frank L. Engel, *Departments of Medicine and Physiology, Duke University, Durham, North Carolina*

WE HAVE BEEN ASKED to open this symposium on the effect of ACTH and cortisone upon infection and resistance by discussing some aspects of the role of the adrenal cortex in intermediary metabolism. Although it had been suspected for some time that the adrenal cortex has an influence upon intermediary metabolism, the basis for our modern concepts concerning this function lies in the report of Long, Katzin, and Fry in 1940 (1), a study with which I am sure you are all thoroughly familiar. Since then a vast amount of investigation has been done in this area. It is obviously impossible for me to review even the most salient details of this work in the time available; nor do I think it would be justifiable to do so before this group, even if time permitted, since most of it is so well known to you. I believe that it will be more profitable to discuss certain working concepts concerning the possible mechanisms by which the adrenal cortex, as well as other endocrine glands, intervene in intermediary metabolism. While it is true that the intensive study of the metabolic actions of the adrenal cortex has not yet yielded to us the information necessary to establish precisely the function of this gland, nevertheless, it has been possible to crystallize more definite concepts as to how the adrenal cortex and the endocrines fit into the total pattern of the regulatory mechanisms of the body from metabolic studies than from investigation of any of the other body functions known to be influenced by the adrenal cortex. At the same time it is true that Hench and Kendall's discovery of the therapeutic action of cortisone in rheumatoid arthritis and the developments which have resulted from this discovery have opened new vistas for research and have made it only too apparent that a consideration of the function of the adrenal cortex only in terms of intermediary metabolism will limit rather than extend knowledge. As a result of this discovery, many investigators in other fields who previously did not concern themselves with the role of endocrines in their experimental results are now actively engaged in studies in which great emphasis is being placed on the influences of the secretions of one gland, the adrenal cortex. It is essential that these investigators now have an appreciation of certain basic facts and concepts of endocrinology. On the other hand, it is also obvious that those who have been interested in certain narrow aspects of endocrinology need to broaden their own vistas, and thereby help to bridge the gap still existing between the various interests that have centered on the adrenal cortex. This should be a profitable procedure for all of us and should result in a cross-fertilization of knowledge and ideas that ought to yield fruitful results. Our greatest need at the moment is for co-operative investigation which will serve to make a meaningful link between the metabolic and the other aspects of adrenal hormone action.

My approach in this discussion then will be to review certain concepts of hormone function which I consider to be cogent to our mutual problems, to outline briefly the better-known metabolic effects of the adrenal hormones, and finally to present some data which may serve to link metabolism and function in relation to certain aspects of infection and resistance.

The most basic concept concerning the endocrine glands is that they are pre-eminently concerned with the maintenance of homeostasis. It is now generally recognized that with respect to the control of intermediary metabolism the adrenal cortex acts in conjunction with the secretions of other endocrines to maintain metabolic homeostasis. The state of normal metabolic balance is dependent on the fine adjustment and interplay of the secretions of the anterior pituitary, thyroid, adrenal cortex, and pancreas. In the event of insufficiency or overactivity of one or more of the hormones of these glands a state of disequilibrium results which persists until a new level of adjustment is achieved, but in each case the organism loses in varying degrees its ability to make those rapid metabolic adjustments which are essential to the maintenance of health or even life. The action of hormones in metabolism is strictly regulatory, involving only rates of reactions, no single metabolic action being either initiated, prevented, or even dependent upon hormones. In the absence of the pituitary, the adrenal cortex, and the pancreas, the gross metabolic picture may appear surprisingly normal, but the organism is totally incapable of buffering the effects of even the slightest threat to its precarious equilibrium. Thus, for example, this preparation rapidly develops hypoglycemia when fasting and hyperglycemia after a meal.

While our knowledge of the roles of hormones in metabolism has been derived largely from studies of the effects of either ablation of a given gland or overdosage of a particular hormone, it must always be realized that these are abnormal situations and may not necessarily reflect the physiological action of the hormone. Thus, for example, both thyroid deficiency and thyroid overdosage result in the development of a negative nitrogen balance dependent, however, on different mechanisms (2).

Furthermore, phenomena observed following ablation of a gland or overdosage of a hormone cannot necessarily be interpreted solely in terms of the hormone in question alone. For example, a small dose of insulin may promote protein anabolism, while larger amounts of the same hormone may stimulate protein catabolism. The latter response is part of the compensatory reaction to hypoglycemia and is dependent on the presence of secretions from the adrenal cortex (3). An uncritical investigator could easily attribute all these effects to insulin. Conversely, it is altogether likely that some of the metabolic changes after ablation of a gland may be due to the unopposed action of hormones with antagonistic actions. Thus, in the adrenalectomized animal the possible effects of endogenous insulin and posterior pituitary antidiuretic hormone must be taken into account when considering fasting hypoglycemia and failure of water diuresis, respectively. It should be apparent, then, that caution is necessary in interpreting results from any experiments with adrenalectomized animals or those in which ACTH or cortisone are used in terms of "physiological actions" of the adrenal cortex until all the necessary information is available to make such inferences. And when we speak of physiological actions, it is important to emphasize that the only incontrovertible physiological actions of the adrenal or any other gland are those which result from endogenous secretions of the gland. As has been emphasized by Dwight Ingle (4), even this cannot be defined in exact units. In the case of the adrenal cortex, it is apparent that large amounts of hormone are necessary to maintain homeostasis in the face of stress. In the absence of stress, the same amount of hormone will produce overdosage effects.

Another concept which is particularly pertinent to any discussion of the adrenal cortex is that of the so-called "permissive" action of a hormone, that is, the concept that a hormone is necessary, but not responsible, for a particular response (4). This, of course, will be recognized as simply another way of stating what we said above, namely, that hormones do not initiate or stop any metabolic reactions, but simply modify rates of reactions.

This permissive concept is exemplified best in studies on the response to injury and its relation to the adrenal cortex. It is now well known that the normal organism responds to injury in a fairly characteristic manner, a response which has been referred to by Selye as the "alarm reaction." The features of this reaction which are common to almost all types of bodily insults include a negative nitrogen balance, an impaired carbohydrate tolerance, a tendency to ketosis, a negative potassium and phosphate balance, retention of sodium and chloride, eosinopenia and lymphopenia, dissolution of lymphoid tissue, and thymic atrophy. At the same time, there are evidences of enhanced activity of the pituitary-adrenal axis manifested by ascorbic acid and cholesterol depletion of the adrenal glands, adrenal hypertrophy, elevated levels of blood corticoids, and increased excretion of corticosteroids in the urine. Since none of these changes takes place in the absence of the adrenal cortex and most of them may be reproduced by administration of ACTH, it is understandable that the earlier interpretation seemed very reasonable, that is, that these are direct effects of the hypersecretion of adrenal steroids in response to stressful stimuli. The fallacy of this interpretation was brought out most clearly by the report of Ingle, Ward, and Kuizenga (5), in which it was shown that adrenalectomized rats maintained on a constant dose of adrenal cortical extract which itself had no appreciable effect on nitrogen excretion responded to a leg fracture with a negative nitrogen balance which was quite as impressive as that in the controls with normal adrenals. Under these experimental conditions no change in adrenal steroid level could occur, and hence it was concluded that the hormones of the adrenal cortex are necessary, but not responsible, for this feature of the response to injury. These results on nitrogen metabolism have been confirmed under different experimental conditions (6-7) and have been extended to electrolyte metabolism (8) to the lymphoid tissue response (9), as well as to many other aspects of the response to injury and of adrenal hormone action (6).

10 ADRENAL CORTEX IN INTERMEDIARY METABOLISM

They point out the difficulty of distinguishing those phenomena which may truly be attributed to hormone action from those phenomena which are part of the reaction to stress, but are, nevertheless, dependent on the presence of adrenal hormones for their initiation and maintenance.

The metabolic reactions whose rates are known or suspected to be influenced by adrenal-hormone action or deficiency are summarized in the diagram below indicating rates of reaction by the size of arrows and concentrations by the height of the columns, and these are compared in normal, adrenalectomized, and animals receiving an overdose

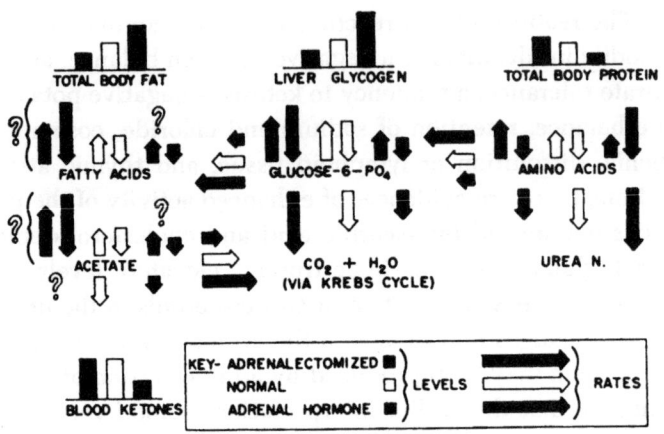

THE ADRENAL CORTEX AND INTERMEDIARY METABOLISM

of adrenal hormone. The size of arrows and columns is entirely arbitrary, and it is not to be inferred that these represent accurately quantitative relationships. Only gross over-all steps in the interconversion of carbohydrate, protein, and fat are indicated, without any attempt either to indicate all the intermediary steps or to pinpoint any possible single site of action of the hormone. It is to be understood that other hormones are involved in this scheme and that by "normal" we refer to the circumstances in which there exists a proper balance between the secretions of all the hormones concerned with intermediary metabolism. This figure emphasizes the continuity of intermediary metabolism, namely, that it is difficult to affect any one part without modifying reactions elsewhere. No attempt will be made to document all the changes to be described. References may be found elsewhere (6, 10–13).

ADRENAL CORTEX IN INTERMEDIARY METABOLISM

We may begin by considering the right side of the graph, that is, protein and amino acid metabolism. Since the report of Long, Katzin, and Fry (1) it has been known that nitrogen excretion may be increased when there has been adrenal-hormone overdosage and decreased when there is adrenal insufficiency. Studies on the protein content of the carcass and of individual tissues, such as lymphoid tissue, thymus, and skin, indicate that these tissues contain less protein than normal in animals treated with adrenal hormone, while in the adrenalectomized animal the relative content of protein and water is greater than is normal in the carcass and in lymphoid tissue. Studies in epiphyseal bone and hair growth in adrenalectomized and in adrenal-hormone-treated animals suggest that protein anabolism (the arrow pointing upward) is increased in the former and decreased in the latter, since these tissues do not ordinarily undergo catabolism. The negative nitrogen balance in the fasted animal receiving adrenal hormones has generally been thought of in terms of increased protein catabolism. Confirmation that both anabolism and catabolism are influenced in the directions indicated has come from studies with N^{15} labeled "amino acids." The overall effect of adrenal-hormone overdosage is to inhibit growth, but the reverse is not necessarily true in the adrenalectomized animal, as the latter's ability to grow is limited by its poor appetite. And finally it should be noted that these effects of adrenal hormone on protein metabolism may be modified considerably by nutritional factors, for a sufficient intake of carbohydrate may sharply decrease or even abolish the negative nitrogen balance from adrenal-hormone overdosage (6).

The changes in amino acid metabolism consequent to adrenal-hormone action are reflected in the rates of urea formation and excretion and in gluconeogenesis, as indicated by the arrows below and to the left of "amino acids." Whether an action of adrenal is exerted at the level of deamination of amino acids has been the subject of considerable debate, having been both denied and affirmed. If there is such an action, it may still be secondary to changes in carbohydrate metabolism, particularly in relation to the Krebs cycle, since, although it is not apparent from this chart, the glycogenic amino acids are converted to glucose only after transformation to the smaller intermediaries.

The change in gluconeogenesis from amino acids noted above is reflected in elevated levels of liver glycogen and blood sugar after adrenal-hormone overdosage, while the reverse is found in the case of the adrenalectomized animal. Evidence for an increased formation of glycogen from nonglucose precursors in the former circumstance and a decrease in the adrenalectomized animal has been obtained by Hastings with the aid of C^{14} labeled "intermediaries." On the other hand, it has been found by a similar technique that the increased liver glycogen levels after adrenal hormone are not associated with an increased rate of conversion of glucose to glycogen, but that actually this rate is less than normal. At the same time, glycogen breakdown is less, so that a net accumulation of liver glycogen may occur. In the adrenalectomized animal the reverse is true, that is, there is an increased synthesis of liver glycogen from glucose, but an even greater breakdown, so that there is a net loss of glycogen. Data from a variety of sources indicate that glucose utilization, probably by way of the Krebs cycle, is increased in the adrenalectomized animal and decreased after adrenal-hormone overdosage, while Welt and Wilhelmi's (14) data suggest the same for the conversion of carbohydrate to fat. Since the adrenalectomized animal which is exhibiting an increased conversion of carbohydrate to fat may at the same time lose body fat, it seems likely that fat breakdown may also be enhanced so that the net effect is the loss of body fat. The opposite appears to be the case during adrenal-hormone overdosage, with net accumulation of fat. These data concerning fat metabolism are still tentative, if not controversial, and are complicated by such observations as those of Altman and others (15) who report a synergistic effect of insulin and cortisone in increasing fat synthesis from carbohydrate in liver, while Balmain and his coworkers (16) describe antagonistic effects of cortisone and insulin on fatty-acid synthesis from labeled acetate in mammary gland tissue, insulin having a stimulating effect, and cortisone an inhibitory one. The studies of Brady, Lukens, and Gurin (17) likewise imply an accelerated synthesis of fatty acids from acetate in liver slices in the absence of the adrenal cortex and its inhibition by cortisone. It is apparent that no certain statements can be made as yet about the role of the adrenal in this aspect of metabolism.

Similarly controversial and unsettled is the question of ketone metabolism and the adrenal cortex. It is widely stated in textbooks and elsewhere that adrenal-hormone overdosage is associated with ketosis. However, Kinsell and his coworkers have shown that both ACTH and cortisone inhibit fasting ketosis in man (18). We have confirmed this in rats during both their fasting and cold stress produced with cortisone and hydrocortisone and have further shown that the previously reported ketosis from ACTH in rats is probably the result of a contaminant, since it can be induced as readily in adrenalectomized rats as in normal rats (19). The latter observation points out the need for caution in interpreting results from experiments with ACTH solely in terms of the effects of adrenal cortical stimulation.

The diagram and the accompanying discussion have outlined the ways in which the adrenal cortex seemingly modifies metabolic reactions. However, it should be recalled that at every point where we have indicated that directly or indirectly the influence of the adrenal cortex is apparent, the impact of other hormones can also be demonstrated. They function in an interlocking manner, any two hormones having both synergistic and antagonistic actions to one another in different phases of intermediary metabolism, resulting in the normal organism in smooth shifts in metabolism to meet the demands of the moment and maintain homeostasis. It is hard to ignore the possibility that the same may be true with regard to those other actions of hormones which have become particularly apparent in recent studies on ACTH and cortisone.

At this time, we might appropriately inquire as to the relations between these metabolic effects of the adrenal cortex and the more recently described tissue and other effects influenced by this gland. In my opinion it can be stated without equivocation that so far it has not been possible to demonstrate any meaningful connection between the known metabolic effects of the adrenal hormones and their therapeutic effectiveness. Yet it is hard to believe that the two are totally dissociated or that there is no relation between the physiological actions of the adrenal cortex in metabolism and the tissue reactions to injury, and so forth. It is in this area that the greatest need exists for co-operative effort between those interested in metabolism and those studying other aspects of adrenal function. Several possible links are suggested. Certainly it appears that the metabolic response to injury noted earlier is meaningful, for when it fails to occur, as in the adrenalectomized animal, not only is the metabolic response deficient, fatal hypoglycemia frequently being the outcome, but the tissues' response is also abnormal. This particular metabolic pattern, which is dependent on the presence of adrenal hormone, is apparently necessary, then, in order that certain of the normal tissue-defense mechanisms may develop fully. At the same time, since we know that the normal defense reaction accompanies stress, while adrenal-hormone overdosage actually lowers some of the defense mechanisms (that is, decreases resistance to bacterial invasion), it would seem likely that other hormones, not only the adrenal cortex, are involved in the normal response to injury.

When we consider demonstrable links between endocrines, metabolism, and function in regard to resistance and infection, we have few data to support us. In the past, interest has been focused on lymphoid tissue, including antibody production, as a result of the studies of Dougherty and White, but this has proven to be a most controversial subject, as will be apparent from later papers in this symposium. Other studies have been directed toward connective-tissue function and metabolism, including observations of certain enzymes, such as hyaluronidase. Recently Dr. Samuel P. Martin, in the Department of Medicine at Duke University, has been approaching this problem by carrying out correlative studies on the function and metabolism of human leukocytes in vitro as influenced by hormones and injury. These studies will be reported in detail at a future date, but preliminary results are shown in the table. In this investigation the oxygen consumption, lactate

EFFECT OF HORMONES ON LEUKOCYTE METABOLISM IN VITRO
(By Dr. S. P. Martin)

	QO_2	Q Lactate	Q Glucose	pH
Compounds E and F 10 gamma/cc	N	−	−	+
Diabetic	?	N	−	?
Insulin 0.1–0.001 u/cc	?	N	N	N
Diabetic with insulin 0.1–0.001 u/cc	?	+	+	?
Endotoxin (Ps. Aerugonosa) 0.5–0.005 gamma/cc (Baxter)	−	+	+	−
Endotoxin + E and F	N	N	N	N

production, glucose utilization, and change in pH of human leukocytes in a phosphate medium containing glucose were studied for several hours. Compared to the normal, incubation with 10 micrograms of cortisone or hydrocortisone per milliliter of cell suspension resulted in no change in oxygen consumption, decreased lactate production, decreased glucose utilization, while the pH of the medium was greater than that of the control at the end of the incubation. Leukocytes from untreated diabetic patients showed a normal lactate production, but decreased glucose utilization. Insulin had no effect on normal cells, but increased the lactate production and glucose utilization of leukocytes from diabetic patients to levels above normal. Cell injury by various endotoxins depressed oxygen consumption and increased both lactate production and glucose utilization, with concomitant fall in pH. Cortisone and hydrocortisone added to the cell suspension three hours prior to the toxins completely prevented the metabolic effects of injury. Martin has also conducted studies on the effects of disease and hormones on leukocyte migration and phagocytosis. The results of all these studies suggest that hormones may play an important role in leukocyte function and that this may eventually be correlated with metabolic changes in these cells. It is from studies of this sort that we hope to achieve an understanding of the role of hormones in the all-important link between cellular function and metabolism.

I will close, then, with the plea that in our enthusiasm for the study of the remarkable effects of ACTH and cortisone, we shall not forget that the adrenal is only one of a set of glands concerned in homeostasis and that with regard to metabolism, at least, it is not possible to divorce the effects of any one gland from that of all others and that all in turn are modified by nonendocrine factors. I need only call to your attention the recent report by Meites that aureomycin and vitamin B_{12} prevent completely thymic atrophy resulting from cortisone in rats on a B_{12} deficient diet to indicate the complexity of the situation (20). We must maintain our perspective and at all times attempt to distinguish between effects of hormones which are physiological and effects which are pharmacological, as well as between effects which are direct and those which are indirect manifestations of hormone action.

REFERENCES

1. Long, C. N. H., B. Katzin, and E. Fry, The adrenal cortex and carbohydrate metabolism, *Endocrinology*, 1940, 26:309.
2. Rupp, J., K. E. Paschkis, and A. Cantarow, Influence of thyroxine on protein metabolism, *Endocrinology*, 1949, 44:449.
3. Engel, F. L., Studies on the nature of the protein catabolic response to adrenal cortical extract; accentuation by insulin hypoglycemia, *Endocrinology*, 1949, 45:170.

4. Ingle, D. J., The functional interrelationship of the anterior pituitary and the adrenal cortex, *Ann. Int. Med.*, 1951, 35:652.
5. Ingle, D. J., E. O. Ward, and M. H. Kuizenga, The relationship of the adrenal glands to changes in urinary non-protein nitrogen following multiple fractures in the force-fed rat, *Am. J. Physiol.*, 1947, 149:510.
6. Engel, F. L., A consideration of the roles of the adrenal cortex and stress in the regulation of protein metabolism, *Recent Progress in Hormone Research*, 1951, 6:277.
7. ——— On the nature of the interdependence of the adrenal cortex, nonspecific stress and nutrition in the regulation of nitrogen metabolism, *Endocrinology*, 1952, 50:462.
8. Ingle, D. J., R. C. Meeks, and D. E. Thomas, The effect of fractures upon urinary electrolytes in non-adrenalectomized rats and in adrenalectomized rats treated with adrenal cortex extract, *Endocrinology*, 1951, 49:703.
9. Herlant, M., Condition, through stress, of the action of corticoids on lymphoid organs, *Proc. Soc. Exp. Biol. & Med.*, 1950, 73:399.
10. Ingle, D. J., The biologic properties of cortisone, *J. Clin. Endocrinology*, 1950, 10:1312.
11. Engel, F. L., Role of the adrenal cortex in intermediary metabolism, *Am. J. Med.*, 1951, 10:556.
12. ——— Relationships between the adrenal cortex and protein metabolism, in Protein Metabolism, Hormones and Growth; a Symposium, Rutgers University Press, New Brunswick, N.J., 1953, p. 34.
13. ——— Pituitary and adrenal glands, *Ann. Rev. of Physiol.*, 1953, 15:397.
14. Welt, I. D., and A. E. Wilhelmi, The effect of adrenalectomy and of the adrenocorticotrophic and growth hormones on the synthesis of fatty acids, *Yale J. Biol. Med.*, 1951, 23:99.
15. Altman, K. I., L. L. Miller, and C. G. Bly, The synergistic effect of cortisone and insulin on lipogenesis in the perfused rat liver as studied with -C^{14}-acetate, *Arch. Biochem.*, 1951, 31:329.
16. Balmain, J. F., S. J. Folley, and F. F. Glascock, Inhibition of fatty acid synthesis in rat mammary gland slices by cortisone in vitro and its antagonism by insulin, *Nature*, 1952, 169:447.
17. Brady, R. O., F. D. W. Lukens, and S. Gurin, Synthesis of radioactive fatty acids in vitro and its hormonal control, *J. Biol. Chem.*, 1951, 193:459.
18. Kinsell, L. W., S. Margen, G. D. Michaels, R. Reiss, F. Frantz, and J. Carbone, Studies in fat metabolism; III: The effect of ACTH, of cortisone, and of other steroid compounds upon fasting-induced hyperketonemia and ketonuria, *J. Clin. Invest.*, 1952, 30:1491.
19. Engel, F. L., and M. G. Engel, Unpublished observations.
20. Meites, J., Changes in nutritional requirements accompanying marked changes in hormone levels, *Metabolism*, 1952, 1:58.

Chapter 3

THE INFLUENCE OF ADRENALECTOMY AND CORTISONE TREATMENT ON CERTAIN ENZYMATIC REACTIONS IN THE RAT

By W. W. UMBREIT, *The Merck Institute for Therapeutic Research, Rahway, N.J.*

THE REMARKABLE EFFECTS of cortisone upon certain diseases has resulted in the search for some explanation of these activities. Naturally, too, some explanation is sought in the field of enzymes, since it is in this area that rather remarkable progress has been made in studies on the "mode of action" of a variety of substances. Of course, hormones have been studied in terms of their enzymatic effects, but on the whole the results have not been striking. Nevertheless, a sufficient number of studies are now available, and in retrospect certain things are now apparent which were not obvious when the studies were begun. I propose to review these briefly; they are admittedly somewhat confusing when considered *en masse*, but such a review is more or less necessary as a backdrop to an analysis of what enzymatic studies have so far found out about the action of the hormones and for an evaluation of what enzyme studies may be expected to contribute to this problem.

Almost all cases are those in which one measures the level of a specific enzyme in the tissue. Here certain facts ought to be recognized.

1. The quantity of a given enzyme in a tissue may not be exactly measurable, and the results obtained are dependent, naturally, upon the method used for measurement. The development of quantitative assay methods for specific enzymes is not as simple a task as has been assumed.

2. The enzymatic complement of a cell is not necessarily a constant matter; it can at times be varied by external influence. For example, the succinoxidase content of the liver of the rat may be markedly depleted by placing the animal on a protein free diet for a few days.

For these reasons one must be wary of alleged changes in the enzyme content of tissues. However, some changes have been observed. Whether or not they are adequate to establish a pattern of response is up to your judgment. I will first describe what is in the literature and give you a brief, if somewhat confusing, summary. I am going to do this for two reasons: (1) To show you what the data are like, hoping that somewhere we may strike a chord of response—that somewhere in this welter of confusion one or more of you may be able to discern a pattern; (2) to illustrate some principles which may possibly emerge: principles that I think may be true of the action of the hormones on enzymes. I am not sure that they are true, however, so first I shall assemble the bricks, and then use those with which I can build a house.

I have confined myself to adrenal steroids, including others only if they affect the same system. For other steroids somewhat comparable types of effects are observed. It is to be understood that all of the following data were obtained by treating the whole animal in the manner described, and then studying the tissue. Experience has shown that this is a very poor approach. The mode of action of vitamins and of antibiotics, insofar as we know them, was not (with one exception) discovered this way, and even that one exception (B_1) was only certain in the animal because of simultaneous studies on bacteria. So far our penetration into the mode of action of such agents has been through studies of bacterial metabolism where the reaction involved was located, followed by confirmatory observations on the animal. But with hormones it is obviously different, and there probably lies the crux of the experimental problem.

That is, the enzyme chemist's reputation for solving problems of "mode of action" rests on studies on vitamins and antibiotics, as well as upon intermediary metabolism. In the case of the hormones he is deprived, by the very nature of the problem, of two of his best tools: (*a*) a microbial system and (*b*) in vitro effects related to in vivo action. I am not sure that a microbial system is absolutely necessary, it just happens that so far one has always been available and that the real advances have come from the study of the microorganism.

Let us briefly examine the effects of adrenalectomy on certain tissue enzymes and their reactions to certain steroids.

Arginase is an enzyme which splits arginine to ornithine and urea. It occurs in liver (best), mammary gland, testes, kidney, and intestinal mucosa. In the liver arginase is subject to several outside influences: sex, age, prolonged fast, and so forth. Hypophysectomy decreases it markedly (1–2); ACTH increases it in normal and hypophysectomized animals, while growth hormone decreases it. Adrenalectomy reduces arginase more than hypophysectomy (1-2). The enzyme could be increased in normal, adrenalectomized, or hypophysectomized animals by corticosterone, 11-dehydrocorticosterone, or cortisone. After treatment with cortisone there is no increase until the protein catabolic effect has worn off (3). DOC has no effect, but DOC and testosterone increase it (4). Estrogens and androgens have no effect. It is decreased by thyrotropic hormone (1) and thyroxine (5).

In the kidney, castration causes an increase in arginase activity per unit weight, but not in total amount, since the castration decreases kidney weight (6-10). The steroids producing kidney hypertrophy (androgens, testosterone, methyltestosterone, and testosterone propionate) increase the absolute arginase content. In the mammary gland, arginase is decreased on adrenalectomy (11) and not restored by adrenal cortical steroids, although lactation is improved.

While the phosphatases are a family of enzymes, the type with which we shall deal here are the phosphomonoesterases, hydrolyzing the orthophosphate monoesters, since in essence they are the only ones which have been studied in relation to adrenal function. But among the phosphomonoesterases we have at least four enzymes which are isodynamic; that is, they catalyze the same reaction, but at different pH's. A simple separation of "acid" and "alkaline" phosphatase is no longer possible, since there are at least three "acid" phosphatases. However, the actual measurements simplify the picture, since only one of the acid phosphatases is normally measured.

Turning first to "alkaline phosphatase," it is especially high in intestinal mucosa, kidney cortex, lactating mammary gland, and lymphoid tissue and lower in liver or brain. Upon adrenalectomy this enzyme decreases in the intestinal mucosa (12) and increases on ACE or cortisone treatment. In the kidney, adrenalectomy decreases alkaline phosphatase (13) which in the rat is restored by salt or DOC (14). Further, in the kidney the administration of testosterone, androsterone, and various derivatives to castrated mice causes kidney hypertrophy and a decrease in alkaline phosphatase (15), with increase in acid phosphatase. In liver and intestinal mucosa these two enzymes are not affected by this treatment. Adrenalectomy of male rats decreases the alkaline phosphatase of the kidney. With testosterone propionate there is a partial return to normal, but castration causes a similar decrease, which is not restored by testosterone, but is restored by estradiol and diethylstilbestrol. Thyroidectomy (or antithyroids) decrease it in kidneys. In the mammary gland upon the onset of lactation, alkaline phosphatase increases it (16).

The alkaline phosphatase of the serum (which is the predominant phosphatase in serum) is apparently derived by diffusion from various tissues, possibly predominantly from the liver. Upon adrenalectomy in the rat or the dog, the enzyme does not decrease appreciably, sometimes increases, but on treatment of either the adrenalectomized animal or the normal animal with cortisone, the alkaline phosphatase rises markedly in both species (14, 17). It is still a moot problem as to whether this is the result of lymphoid disintegration, since lymphoid tissue is rich in this enzyme and, of course, is subject to breakdown by cortisone. Testosterone propionate has no effect (17). Bone alkaline phosphatase is decreased by ACE and corticosterone and increased by DOC (18).

The acid phosphatase is widely distributed, but in much lower quantities than is the alkaline phosphatase. The human prostate is high in it, and it is appreciable in liver and spleen. It is curious that in the prostate it is present only in man and the higher apes and virtually absent from this organ in other mammals. As mentioned, the administration of testosterone and so forth to castrated mice causes a marked increase in kidney acid phosphatase (with a decrease in alkaline phosphatase). Adrenalectomy increases serum acid phosphatase in the rat, which is decreased by administration of testosterone propionate (17).

About three years ago there was a considerable flurry of interest in relation to the peptidases of human and animal serum. It was suggested that the presence of peptidases in the sera might be caused by the liberation of the enzymes in the course of disintegration of lymphoid tissue. It was then reported (19) that in mice injection of ACE or ACTH considerably increased serum peptidase, from which it was suggested that this resulted from liberation from lymphoid cells. However, in human beings ACTH did not increase serum peptidase in spite of a large turnover in lymphocytes, and, indeed, when the earlier experiments were repeated by others (20–21) it was found that serum peptidase was not related to adrenal steroids, ACTH, or lymphoid tissue, but that the effects were caused by disintegration of the erythrocytes, which are potent sources of these enzymes.

The D-amino acid oxidase of the liver is decreased on adrenalectomy and restored to normal by cortisone (22–23). With respect to the kidney, there are two reports: one that adrenalectomy or cortisone treatment has no effect (23) and the other that the enzyme is decreased on adrenalectomy (22). The studies differ in the methods used for measurement, and since I was responsible for one of them (23) I naturally think that cortisone and adrenalectomy have no effect on kidney D-amino acid oxidase. The monamine oxidase of the liver is higher in the adult male than in the female, but in the male it may be decreased to the female level by cortisone treatment; adrenalectomy has no effect (24). The proline oxidase system of the kidney, but not that of the liver, is decreased on adrenalectomy and restored to normal by cortisone treatment (25). Liver catalase is decreased on adrenalectomy (26).

This rapid review is confusing, but it serves the purpose of illustrating the experimental facts. There are unquestionably other enzymes which are altered by these treatments, for I do not claim complete coverage of the literature, and doubtless many other publications will appear after further study. However, a sufficient pattern is even now available to permit some degree of evaluation of this type of approach. To the best of my knowledge, all of these effects are observable only by treatment of the whole animal. There are no known in vitro responses. Furthermore, all of the effects cited require at least a day for development but usually several days of treatment are necessary. It seems obvious that the hormones are not acting as coenzymes. Cortisone does not act rapidly on the systems mentioned. Turning specifically to cortisone, one may summarize some of the information available in the

Behavior of the Enzyme after Adrenalectomy [a]

Organ	Arginase	Alkaline Phosphatase	Proline Oxidase	D-amino Acid Oxidase
Liver	Is decreased −		Is unaltered −	Is decreased +
Kidney	Is unaltered +	Is decreased	Is decreased +	Is unaltered −
Mammary gland	Is decreased −			
Serum		Unaltered +		

[a] + indicates that the level of enzyme is increased by cortisone treatment; − indicates that cortisone has no effect.

table. Here a curious specificity is evident. A given treatment may have one effect upon an enzyme in one tissue, but another effect on the same enzyme in another tissue. Furthermore, there are all possible combinations evident in this table. And finally, it does not demonstrate another fact evident in the previous papers cited, namely, that a given enzyme may be under the control of one steroid hormone in one tissue, but another hormone in another. For example, alkaline phosphatase is lowered on adrenalectomy in the intestinal mucosa and restored by cortisone (12), but it is not affected by testosterone (15). In the kidney, adrenalectomy also lowers alkaline phosphatase, which is restored by saline, DOC, or testosterone (14–15). Certainly we are not obtaining a clear picture of the mode of action of cortisone from data of this type.

Yet in a general way some principles may be deduced from this confusion and contradiction. Using only the two enzymes proline oxidase and D-amino acid oxidase, one may first note the curious tissue specificity. Proline oxidase is under the control of cortisone in the kidney, but not in the liver. D-amino acid oxidase is under the control of cortisone in the liver, but not in the kidney. Various other enzymes appear to show the same phenomenon of tissue specificity. If we look for a general term to describe this tissue specificity we might employ the term "target organ." And this represents merely an extension of the concept of target organ to the tissue enzyme level.

Turning again to proline oxidase and D-amino acid oxidase, upon adrenalectomy the activity of these enzymes in their respective target tissues drops, not to exactly the same extent, but roughly in the same order of magnitude. But there is a residual activity of about one fourth to one half which remains, in the absence of cortisone, at the same level for months. It seems to me that this is an expression of the concept that a hormone does not initiate a reaction, but only affects its rate or extent. For both enzymes cortisone restores activity to normal, but more cortisone does not increase the level beyond the normal level. This is not true of all the other enzymes cited. This is an expression of the principle that a hormone only acts within certain limits.

And finally, in all known cases the hormone is active only when supplied to the animal and controls the amount of enzyme present. This, too, is an expression of the notion that the hormones are the chemical messengers of the body.

These you will recognize as reasonably basic principles of endocrinology. It is curious that one is able to derive them from studies on the tissue enzymes, although these principles were known before anyone studied tissue enzymes. Studies on the enzymatic composition of the tissues have not clarified the underlying causes; the mode of action of the adrenal hormones remains as mysterious as ever.

REFERENCES

1. Fraenkel-Conrat, H., M. E. Simpson, and H. M. Evans, Effect of hypophysectomy and of purified pituitary hormones on the liver arginase activity of rats, *Am. J. Physiol.*, 1943, 138:439.
2. ——— Influence of adrenalectomy and of adrenocortical steroids on liver arginase, *J. Biol. Chem.*, 1943, 147:99.
3. Kochakian, C. D., Recent studies on the *in vivo* and *in vitro* effect of hormones on enzymes, *Ann. N.Y. Acad. Sci.*, 1951, 54:534.
4. ——— Macy Conference Metabolic Aspects of Convalescence, Including Bone and Wound Healing—6th Meeting, Feb. 11–12, 1944, p. 13.
5. Lightbody, H. D., E. Witt, and A. Kleinman, Variations in arginase concentration in livers of white rats caused by thyroxine administration, *Proc. Soc. Exp. Biol. & Med.*, 1941, 46:472.
6. Kochakian, C. D., The effect of castration and various steroids on the arginase activity of the tissues of the mouse, *J. Biol. Chem.*, 1944, 155:579.
7. ——— The effect of dose and nutritive state on kidney arginase after steroid stimulation, *J. Biol. Chem.*, 1945, 161:115.
8. Kochakian, C. D., and C. E. Stettner, Effect of testosterone propionate and growth hormone on the arginase and phosphatases of the organs of the mouse, *Am. J. Physiol.*, 1948, 155:262.
9. Kochakian, C. D., E. E. Garber, and M. N. Bartlett, Effect of estrogen alone and in combination with testosterone on the body and organ weights and the arginase and phosphatases of the organs of the mouse, *Am. J. Physiol.*, 1948, 155:265.
10. Kochakian, C. D., M. N. Bartlett, and J. Moe, Effect of high protein and high carbohydrate diets on the arginase and phosphatases of the liver and kidney of the normal and adrenalectomized rat, *Am. J. Physiol.*, 1948, 154:489.
11. Folley, S. J., and A. L. Greenbaum, Effects of adrenalectomy and of treatment with adrenal cortex hormones on the arginase and phosphatase levels of lactating rats, *Biochem. J.*, 1945, 40:46.
12. Kutscher, W., and H. Wüst, Nebennierenrinde und alkalische Phosphatase, *Z. Physiol. Chem.*, 1943, 273:235.
13. ——— Nebenniere und alkalische Phosphatase, *Naturwiss*, 1941, 29:319.
14. Vail, V. N., and C. D. Kochakian, The effect of adrenalectomy, adrenal cortical hormones, and testosterone propionate plus adrenal cortical extract on the "alkaline" and "acid" phosphatases of the liver and kidney of the rat, *Am. J. Physiol.*, 1947, 150:580.

15. Kochakian, C. D., The role of hydrolytic enzymes in some of the metabolic activities of the steroid hormones, *Recent Progress in Hormone Research*, 1947, 1:177.
16. Folley, S. J., and A. L. Greenbaum, Changes in the arginase and alkaline phosphatase contents of the mammary gland and liver of the rat during pregnancy, lactation, and mammary involution, *Biochem. J.*, 1947, 211:261.
17. Buchwald, K. W., L. Hudson, and J. Bellanca, The biochemical effects of sex hormones in adrenalectomized rats, *Endocrinology*, 1950, 47:228.
18. Williams, H. L., and E. M. Watson, Influence of hormones upon phosphatase content of rat femurs; I: Effects of adrenal cortical substances and parathyroid extract, *Endocrinology*, 1942, 29:250.
19. Holman, H. R., A. White, and J. S. Fruton, Relation of the adrenal cortex to serum peptidase activity, *Proc. Soc. Exp. Biol. & Med.*, 1947, 65:196.
20. Engel, F. L., and T. B. Schwartz, Adrenal cortex and peptidase activity of rat tissue, *Proc. Soc. Exp. Biol. & Med.*, 1951, 77:615.
21. Schwartz, T. B., and F. L. Engel, The adrenal cortex and serum peptidase activity, *J. Biol. Chem.*, 1949, 180:1047.
22. Jensen, H., and J. L. Gray, The influence of hormones on the amino acid dihydrogenase systems of the liver and kidney, *Ann. N.Y. Acad. Sci.*, 1951, 54:619.
23. Umbreit, W. W., and N. E. Tonhazy, Metabolic action of cortisone: D-amino acid oxidase and apparent creatinine formation, *Arch. Biochem.*, 1951, 32:96.
24. Schweppe, J. S., E. A. Zeller, and G. M. Higgins, Interrelationships between enzymes and hormones; VI: Influence of age, sex, adrenalectomy, and cortisone acetate upon the concentration of monamine oxidase in the livers of white rats, *Proc. Staff Meet. Mayo Clinic*, 1951, 26:371.
25. Umbreit, W. W., and N. E. Tonhazy, The metabolic effects of cortisone; I: The oxidation of proline, *J. Biol. Chem.*, 1951, 191:249.
26. Begg, R. W., and E. F. Reynolds, Effect of adrenalectomy on liver catalase activity in the rat, *Science*, 1950, 111:721.

Chapter 4

THE EFFECT OF CORTICOSTEROIDS UPON LYMPHOID TISSUE

BY WILLIAM E. EHRICH AND JOSEPH SEIFTER, *Graduate School of Medicine, University of Pennsylvania, Philadelphia General Hospital, and Wyeth Institute of Applied Biochemistry*

THE INTERRELATION between adrenals and lymphoid tissue has been apparent for many years. Hyperplasia of the thymus in Addison's disease was observed in 1895 by Star; thymic enlargement following adrenalectomy was noted in 1899 by Boinet (1). That the "status thymicolymphaticus" of Paltauff (2) is caused by hypofunction of the adrenals was recognized in 1924 by Jaffe (3) and by Marine and his associates (4-5). These investigators concluded that the adrenals normally suppress or exert a regulating effect upon thymus and other lymphoid structures.

The rapid involution of thymus and other lymphoid structures following various stresses was first described in 1913 as "crise caryoclasique" by Dustin and in 1921 as "crise hemoclastique" by Widal (1, 6-8). The role of the adrenals in this morphological expression of an "alarm reaction" was first demonstrated in 1936 by Selye (1, 9). Since in adrenalectomized animals involution failed to develop, but it could be induced by injection of cortin, Selye considered increased cortin secretion the cause of the involution (9). Because in adrenalectomized animals only large doses of this extract were effective (1) and steroid hormones other than adrenal corticosteroids elicited a similar effect (10), he also offered an alternative explanation, namely, that the involution was caused by an unknown agent associated with these steroids (9). The observation that thymic involution may be caused by the administration of large doses of cortin was soon confirmed by Carriere and others (11) and Ingle (12).

The effect upon lymphoid tissue of the various corticosteroids and other steroid hormones has subsequently been studied by many investigators. The depression of lymphoid tissue by 11-oxy- and hydroxycorticosteroids (Kendall's compounds *A, B, E* and *F*) was first observed by

Ingle and others (13–15) in intact animals and by Dougherty and White (16–18) in adrenalectomized animals. Desoxycorticosteroids in small doses had no effect on lymphoid tissue, but large doses caused thymic involution in both intact and adrenalectomized animals (19–24). The failure of some investigators (15–18, 25) to confirm these observations can be attributed to inadequate doses (15–18) or improper time intervals (25).

The involuting action on lymphoid tissue of ACTH had been observed previously by Moon (26); that it requires the presence of the adrenals was subsequently demonstrated by Simpson and others (27) and by Dougherty and White (16–18).

Steroid hormones other than adrenal corticosteroids which have been shown to cause thymic involution in both intact and adrenalectomized animals include estrogen (that is, estrone, estradiol, diethylstilbestrol), testosterone (that is, methyl-testosterone, dehydro-iso-androsterone), and to a lesser extent pregnanediol and similar compounds (10, 19, 21, 28–31). Progesterone produced a significant effect only in intact animals (10, 19, 21, 29, 32). Selye and others (21, 29) have pointed out that the effectiveness of these steroids increases with their physiological activity, sexually inert substances causing no thymic involution. The thymus-involuting effect of the sex hormones could be induced only by doses many times larger than those required for their physiological action. It is interesting that the various sex hormones produced also involution of the Leydig cells. According to Selye and Albert (21) this fact almost certainly implicates in this action the anterior pituitary gland.

Gonadotropin also was found to cause thymic involution, but it did so only in the presence of the gonads, suggesting that it acts by stimulating their secretory activity (33).

The morphological changes induced in lymphoid tissue by these various hormones have been described repeatedly. Selye (1, 6) noted edema and distintegration of lymphocytes twenty-four hours after stress or administration of cortin. After forty-eight hours these changes disappeared. The reticuloendothelial cells did not disintegrate, but underwent enlargement. These changes were most marked in the thymus; in lymph nodes and spleen they occurred chiefly in the so-called germinal centers.

A more detailed study of the effect of the adrenal corticosteroids upon lymphoid tissue was made by Dougherty and White (17–18). Edema was pronounced within one hour. "Lymphocytolysis," characterized by shedding of cytoplasm and by pyknosis and karyorrhexis of nuclei, and phagocytosis by macrophages of disintegrating cells, were evident within the first three hours. The intensity of this reaction increased during the following six hours, after which edema subsided and no further disintegration of lymphocytes was observed. The cortex of the thymus and the germinal centers of lymph nodes and spleen were more sensitive than other lymphoid structures. In the germinal centers most of the large pale cells ("large lymphocytes," "lymphoblasts") remained unaffected, but no mitotic figures were seen. After twenty-four to thirty-six hours the appearance of the tissue was normal.

The histological changes following continued daily injections of rats with ACTH have recently been described by Baker and others (34). Lymphocytolysis proceeded throughout the experimental period of twenty-one days. The formation of new lymphocytes was sharply curtailed, as was previously suggested by Yoffey and Baxter (35) and by Robertson (36); mitotic figures were generally absent, and large and medium-size lymphocytes were greatly reduced in number. Baker and others pointed out that the plasma cells were not increased in number as was previously reported by Dougherty and White (37); on the contrary, they were depleted from the lymph nodes if sufficient hormone was given. The latter observation is in agreement with our findings (38).

Depression of the lymphocyte content of the thoracic duct by ACTH was demonstrated by Reinhardt and Li (39) and by Yoffey and others (40). That lymphocytopenia may be caused by 11-oxy- and hydroxycorticosteroids was shown by Dougherty and White (16, 18, 41), Reinhardt and others (42) and Yoffey and Baxter (35). The reduction in the thoracic duct occurred within fifteen to thirty minutes after injection and persisted in most rats for the duration of the experiment (four to ten hours) (39). The depression of the circulating lymphocytes continued for nine hours; thereafter these cells returned to normal (16, 18, 41).

The mechanism of action of the adrenal corticosteroids upon lymphoid tissue has not been elucidated. In vitro studies with isolated lymphocytes led to contradictory results. Dougherty and White (17), adding aqueous adrenal cortical extract to suspensions of rat lymphocytes, found no increased lymphocytolysis. No effect was seen in similar experiments with eschatin and eucortine by Robertson (36), who also used serum of rats injected with these steroids three hours previous to its withdrawal. Negative results were obtained in experiments with compound A by Delaunay and others (43), and in experiments with compound E by Reiss and others (44). The latter found no effect of this compound upon the phenomenon of agglutination of bacteria by antibody-forming plasma cells.

On the other hand, Schreck (45), who studied lymphocytes of rabbit thymus suspensions by means of a safranine method, reported increased disintegration of lymphocytes by compounds B and F twenty-one hours after adding these steroids, while ACTH, DCA, and sex hormones were ineffective. In a subsequent study Schreck (46), employing a color test based on the capacity of cellular suspensions to reduce 2,-6-dichlorophenol indophenol, observed evidence of lymphocytolysis following administration of adrenal cortical extract or 1 gamma percent of cortisone acetate. But even in this experiment lymphocytolysis was noticeable only after seven hours, while in vivo it developed fully two hours after injection. However, Feldman (47), using Schreck's method, reported that adrenal cortical extract had an instantaneous effect upon suspensions of lymphocytes. Immediately after addition of the material 60 percent of the cells were found to be stained; after three hours the figure was 90 percent, and after six hours 100 percent; after six hours only 6 percent were dead in the control preparations. It was noted, however, that compound E had no such effect.

Somewhat different results were obtained when tissue or tissue extracts, instead of washed lymphocytes, were used in vitro. Thus Heilman (48), using a tissue culture method, found that the addition to 1 ml of medium of 1.25 to 60 micrograms of compound E or of similar quantities of compound A caused a slight, but significant, degeneration and inhibition of migration of small and medium-size lymphocytes associated with an increase in the number of large wandering cells (macrophages). Small doses were as effective as large doses. Similarly, Hechter and Johnson (49) observed that the rate of lymphocytolysis in vitro was significantly augmented by 10 mg per ml of medium of adrenal cortical extract if lymphoid tissue homogenates were added. Brain homogenates had a similar effect, while muscle homogenates or homologous serum were ineffective. Desoxycorticosteroids were altogether negative, but sex hormones caused lymphocytolysis even when incubated with serum.

Interesting results were recently reported by Herlant (50). When adrenalectomized rats weighing 150–180 gms were exposed to stress or 0.2 ml of adrenal cortical extract or both, it was found that the extract alone produced little lymphocytolysis, while the two procedures together caused extensive caryclasia. These observations strongly suggest that the steriods act in association with a conditioning factor or cofactor (49–50), as was suspected by Selye as early as 1936 (9). It may well be that this factor is associated with the edema which has been observed so consistently since first described by Selye (1) and later pointed out by Dougherty and White (17). According to Selye (8) the edema may act either by sensitizing the lymphoid tissue or by activating the steroids. It is possible that it is related to the cofactor which appears to operate in the hyperglycemic action of these steroids (8).

The reason why the lymphoid cells are singled out by the steroids is not clear. Hechter and Johnson (49), Schreck (45), and Selye (8) considered responsible their high content in desoxyribose nucleoprotein or the action of desoxyribose nuclease upon this nucleoprotein. It had previously been suggested by us (51) that this affinity may be connected with the high concentration of ribose nucleoprotein contained in their cytoplasm rather than the desoxyribose nucleoprotein of their nuclei.

Our interest in this problem dates back to 1945, when we were looking for a morphological indicator of nonspecific toxicity. It was found that the weight of the thymus offers an indicator (52). Table 1 shows the effect of goitrogenic compounds upon thymus weight as compared with their action upon body weight and their specific effect upon thyroid weight. Doses of compounds which caused depression of thymus weight were regarded as toxic.

Microscopic studies of the thymus of animals treated with toxic doses of drugs revealed that the depression of its weight was caused by lymphocytolysis. Obviously we were dealing with Selye's alarm reaction (7). It was found that lymphocytolysis can easily be graded. Figure 1 shows various grades of lymphocytolysis caused by dibenamine and colchicine. The lymphocytolytic effect of dibenamine is interesting in view of the theory first proposed by Long (53) that epinephrine is responsible for anterior pituitary stimulation caused by stress. If this theory were correct, dibenamine should have neutralized epinephrine and thus prevented lymphocytolysis. Instead, it caused lymphocytolysis by itself (54). However, Figure 2 shows that the epinephrine theory should not be disregarded. It is true that dibenamine does not prevent, but augments the initial phase of lymphocytolysis caused by epinephrine; but it depresses it later. This observation suggests that there may be two phases of lymphocytolysis, namely, an immediate phase, with a peak at two hours, and a later phase, becoming apparent after six hours; the latter may occur only in more severe alarm reactions.

TABLE 1

EFFECTS UPON THYROID, BODY AND THYMUS WEIGHT OF VARIOUS CONCENTRATIONS OF GOITROGENIC COMPOUNDS

	Dose; Percentage in Drinking Water	Number of Rats	Percentage of Body Weight Change per Day	Thyroid Weight, mg/gm	Thymus Weight, mg/gm
Controls	...	40	+6.1	.14	3.3
Thiouracil	.01	4	+8.5	.29	3.3
Thiouracil	.02	4	+8.2	.34	3.25
Thiouracil	.05	8	+6.6	.50	2.8
Propylthiouracil	.01	4	+7.2	.63	2.9
Propylthiouracil	.05	4	+7.5	.56	2.7
Propylthiouracil	.10	4	+6.4	.51	2.3
Propylthiouracil	.25	4	+2.2	.60	1.7
Two aminothiazole	.10	40	+4.4	.36	2.5
Dithane	.05	4	+3.8	.18	2.5
Dithane	.10	4	+3.5	.65	2.3
Dithane	.15	4	+1.6	.71	1.9

From J. Seifter and W. E. Ehrich, Goitrogenic compounds, *J. Pharm. a. Exp. Ther.*, 1948, 92:303.

Figure 3 shows the dependence upon the adrenals of lymphocytolysis caused by stress. One injection of a potent anti-kidney serum causes complete necrosis of the thymus cortex, followed by a marked drop in thymus weight. This is associated with a marked rise in adrenal weight. Adrenalectomized rats also show some augmentation of lymphocytolysis, but this is not severe enough to alter the weight of this organ.

In considering the effect on lymphoid tissue of adrenal corticosteroids, it is to be recognized that there are at least three different lymphoid tissues. These are (1) the diffuse lymphoid tissue of the cortex of thymus and lymph nodes, of the lymph sheaths of the spleen, and of other lymphoid tissues; (2) the so-called germinal centers of lymph nodes, spleen, tonsils, and intestine; and (3) the plasma-cell tissue of the medullary cords of lymph nodes and of the red pulp of the spleen.

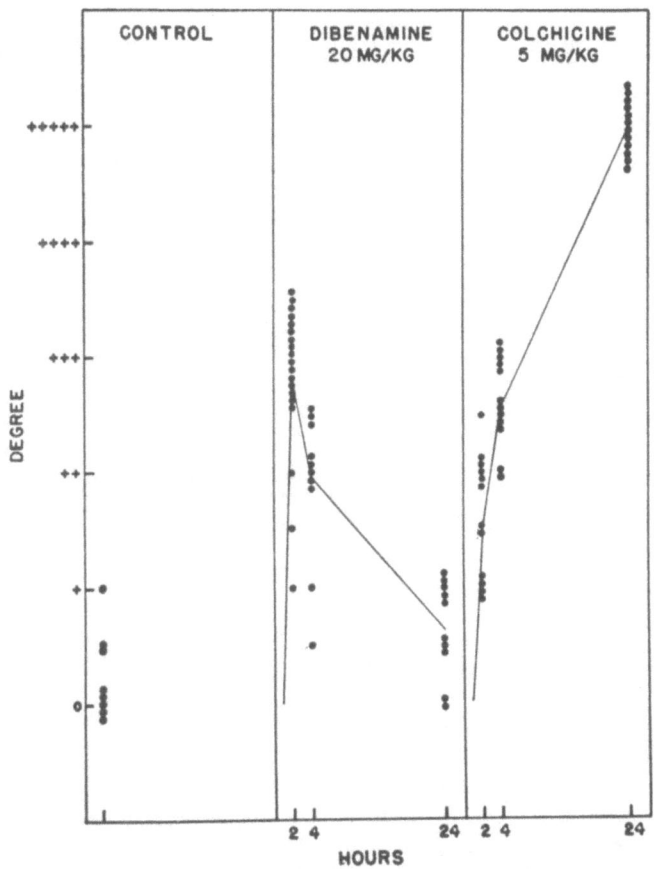

FIGURE 1. LYMPHOCYTOLYSIS IN THYMUS

While diffuse lymphoid tissue is always present, germinal centers and plasma-cell tissue may be present or absent, depending upon certain stimuli. The function of the plasma cells may now be regarded as established. The evidence shows that they are cellular sources of antibodies and other gamma globulins (55). The function of the germinal centers is less known. It is true that they are physiological centers of lymphocytolysis (56), but we do not know whether the large pale lymphoid cells

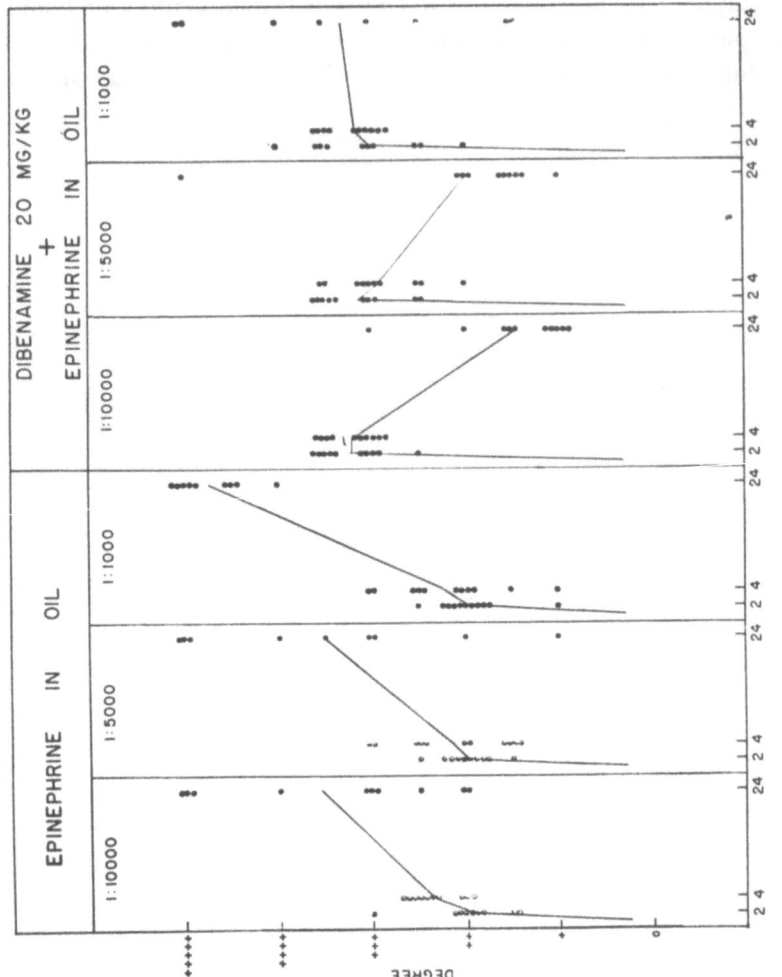

FIGURE 2. LYMPHOCYTOLYSIS IN THYMUS, EPINEPHRINE IN OIL HAVING BEEN GIVEN IN DOSES OF 0.25 ML EVERY HOUR

EFFECT OF CORTICOSTEROIDS

which constitute the bulk of this tissue are lymphoblasts or hemocytoblasts or whether they have special enzymatic functions. The role of the small lymphocytes which constitute the bulk of the diffuse lymphoid tissue will be discussed later.

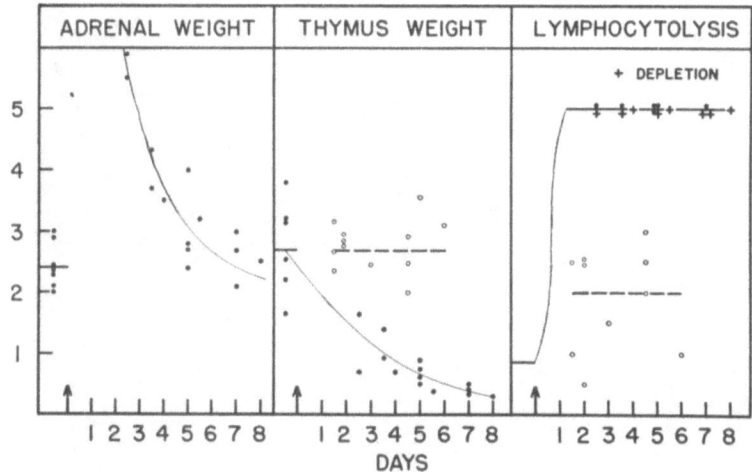

FIGURE 3. EFFECTS OF ANTI-RAT-KIDNEY SERUM IN INTACT (·) AND ADRENALECTOMIZED (○) RATS

These data were collected by Dr. C. Forman and one of the authors during a study of experimental nephrosis. The figures at the left indicate mg/10g of body weight (of adrenals and thymus) and degrees (of lymphocytolysis in the cortex of the thymus); 5 + lymphocytolysis indicates complete necrosis.

Figure 4 shows various degrees of lymphocytolysis of the diffuse lymphoid tissue of the thymus cortex produced by various stresses. It can be seen that many disintegrating lymphocytes have been taken up by phagocytes. Figure 5 is an example of induced plasmocytolysis in medullary cords of lymph nodes. No phagocytosis is seen. Instead, dissolution of cells may be observed. Table 2 shows depression of circulating lymphocytes six hours following intravenous injection of a typhoid vaccine.

Figures 6 and 7 present the effect of 5–10 mg per 100 gm of body weight of cortone and of 50 mg per 100 gm of DCA upon the thymus of intact rats weighing 60–80 gms. While 5–10 mg of cortone had a marked lymphocytolytic effect, though this was less marked than that induced by some stresses employed, 50 mg of DCA caused only mild

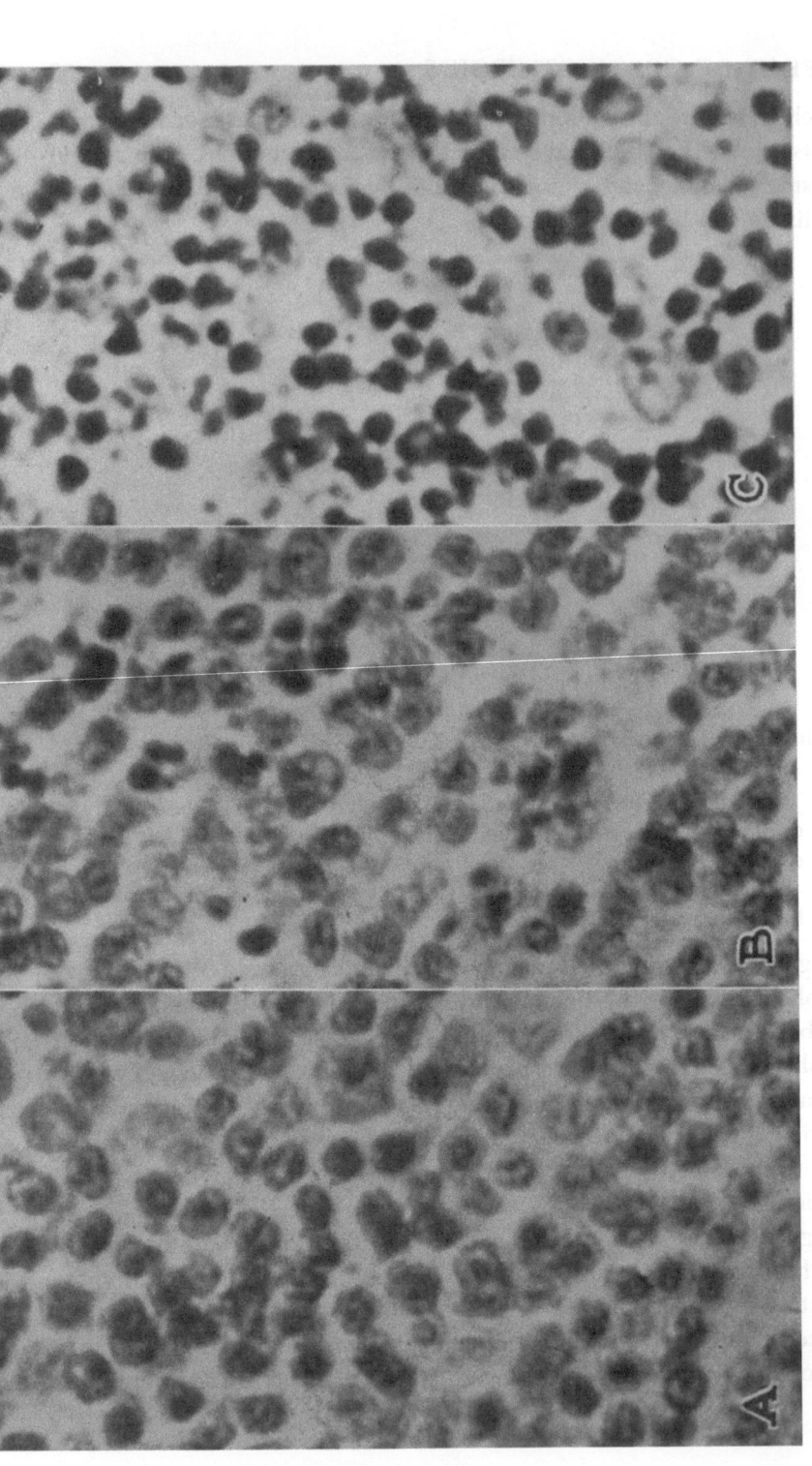

FIGURE 4. CORTEX OF A NORMAL THYMUS IN A YOUNG RAT (A), MODERATE LYMPHOCYTOLYSIS CAUSED BY MILD STRESS (B), AND COMPLETE LYMPHOCYTOLYSIS CAUSED BY MARKED STRESS (C). Note phagocytosis of disintegrating lymphocytes by macrophages. (From W. E. Ehrich, Present state of adrenal cortical hormones, pathological aspects, in Advances in Medicine and Surgery, Saunders, Philadelphia, 1952.)

lymphocytolysis. This is in contrast to ACTH, which has been found to cause complete necrosis of the cortex in doses as small as 0.3 mg per 100 gm (Baker and others; 34). It may be noted that both curves show the biphasic character referred to previously. There was a peak at two hours, and another after six hours, suggesting that lymphocytolysis may be caused by more than one mechanism.

TABLE 2

LEUKOCYTE COUNTS SIX HOURS AFTER ONE INTRAVENOUS INJECTION OF A TYPHOID VACCINE

	B.E.		W.E.		C.F.	
	Control	Six Hrs.	Control	Six Hrs.	Control	Six Hrs.
Neutrophiles	4,902	9,903	6,105	10,248	2,965	11,745
Lymphocytes	3,010	1,049	1,403	1,098	2,239	1,215
Monocytes	430	582	412	732	423	405
Eosinophiles	258	116	330	122	423	135

From W. E. Ehrich, The clinical and pathological significance of the alarm reaction, *J. Phila. Gen. Hosp.*, 1:27, 1950.

Following the administration of 5–10 mg per 100 gm of cortone lymphocytolysis in the germinal centers was only slightly increased, the degree of elevation paralleling that of the diffuse lymphoid tissue of the thymus cortex. This seems to show that lymphocytolysis of the germinal centers will be augmented by adrenal corticosteroids only if given in doses high enough to cause a greater degree of thymic lymphocytolysis than that seen in germinal centers normally.

While lymphocytolysis was easy to grade, plasmocytolysis was difficult to measure. Figure 8 shows our observations in three series of rats treated with formalin, cortisone, or both. The biphasic character of the reaction is seen in all three curves. If severe enough, plasmocytolysis results in depletion of plasma cells, showing that they have a similar susceptibility to adrenal corticosteroids or stress as lymphocytes.

The significance of lymphocytolysis and plasmocytolysis following stress, or the injection of adrenal corticosteroids or sex hormones, is not fully understood. The disintegration of these various cells is obviously associated with liberation and degradation of protein. It has been suggested by Dougherty and White (16) that this process may be instrumental in the gluconeogenic effect of the 11-oxy- and hydroxycorticosteroids, the basis for this action lying not primarily in their influence on the intermediary reactions of carbohydrate formation, but in their

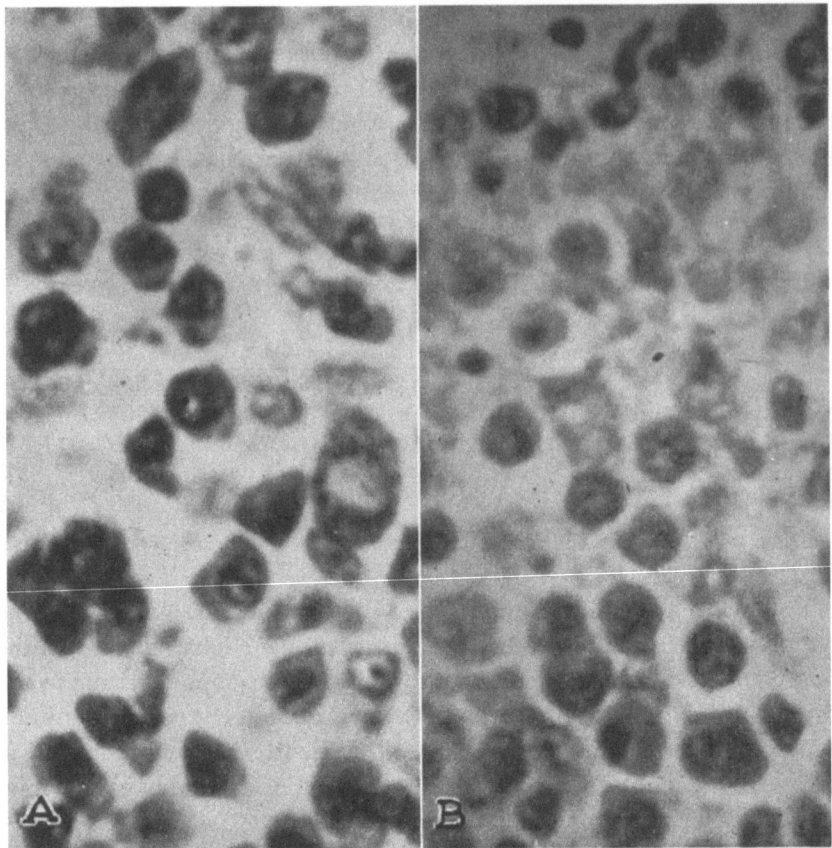

FIGURE 5. PLASMA CELLS IN A LYMPH NODE OF A NORMAL RAT (A) AND CONSIDERABLE PLASMOCYTOLYSIS CAUSED BY MARKED STRESS (B)

Note absence of macrophages. (From W. E. Ehrich, Present state of adrenal cortical hormones, pathological aspects, in Advances in Medicine and Surgery, Saunders, Philadelphia, 1952.)

capacity to supply protein to the sugar-forming tissues. Bergner and Dean (57) have pointed out that this idea tallies with the observation that significant glycogen deposition in the liver following ACTH administration occurs only after eighteen to twenty-four hours, while lymphocytolysis is marked after six hours. This relationship is well illustrated in Figure 9, which shows the effect of 5–10 mg per 100 gm of cortone upon glycogen content of the liver of rats as compared with lymphocytolysis in the thymus cortex.

EFFECT OF CORTICOSTEROIDS

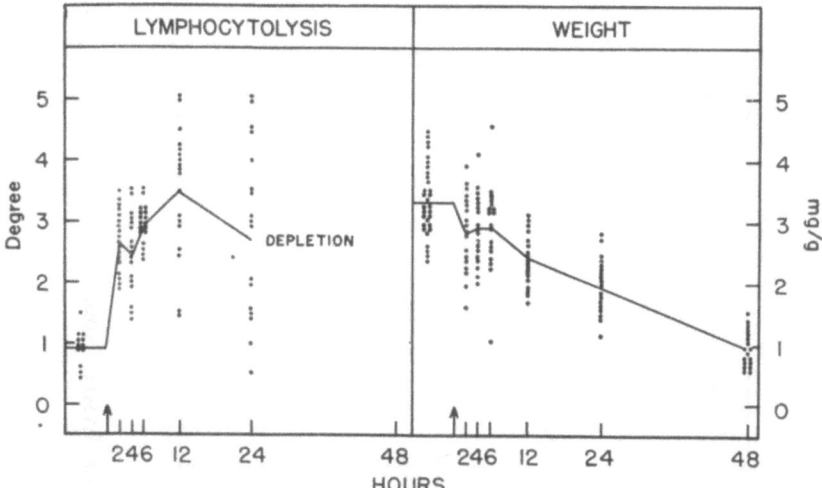

FIGURE 6. EFFECT OF 5–10MG/100G OF CORTISONE UPON THYMUS OF RATS

The disintegration of plasma cells may possibly lead to liberation of antibodies and other gamma globulins, as was first claimed by Dougherty, White, and Chase (17–18, 58–59) though these authors referred to lymphocytes rather than plasma cells. The failure of subsequent investigators to confirm these investigations does not necessarily invalidate the previous conclusion, because the later investigators may have

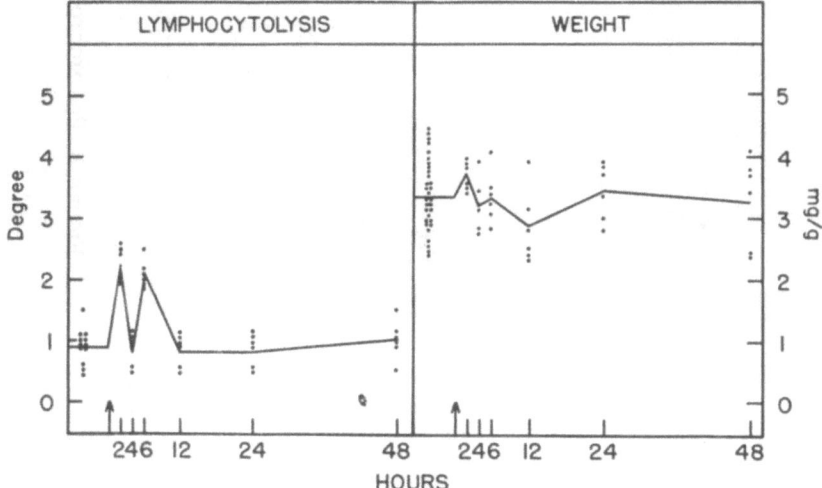

FIGURE 7. EFFECT OF 50MG/100G OF DCA UPON THYMUS OF RATS

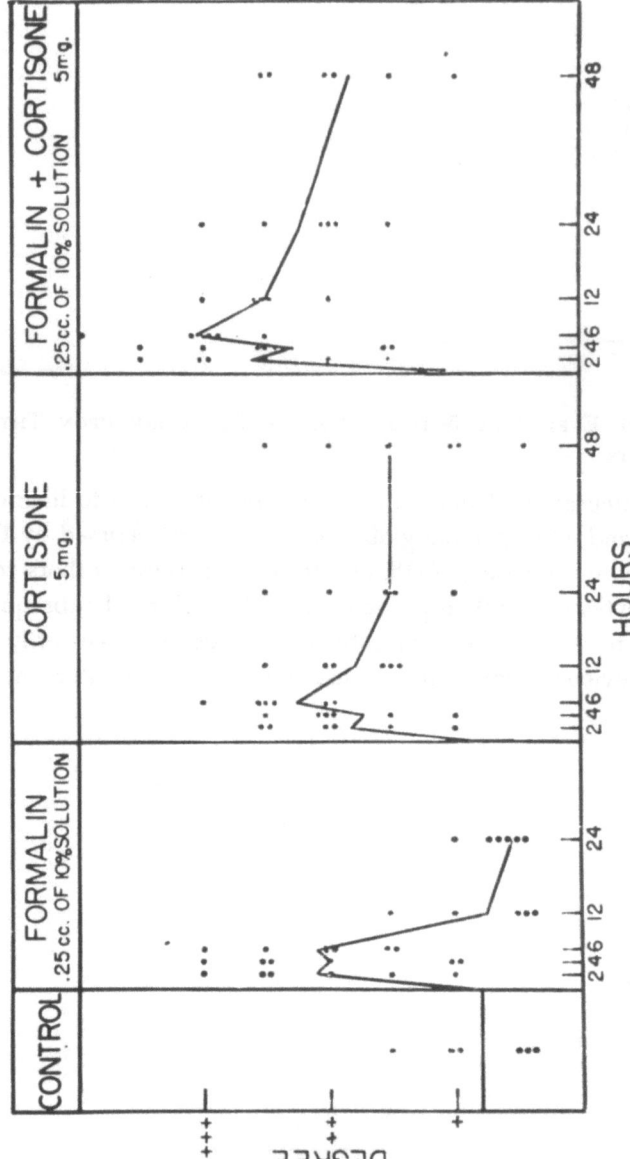

FIGURE 8. PLASMOCTOLYSIS IN MEDULLARY CORDS OF LYMPH NODES

EFFECT OF CORTICOSTEROIDS 39

dealt with animals which contained fewer plasma cells or less antibody in these cells, or they may have used stimuli which were not strong enough to cause dissolution of these cells.

Lymphocytolysis and plasmocytolysis also result in liberation of nucleic acids and their split products. In fact, lymphocytes consist largely of nucleoproteins. The thymus of young rats has been found to contain 114–135 mg per 100 gm of fresh tissue of ribose nucleic acid phosphorus, a quantity which is surpassed only by the amount con-

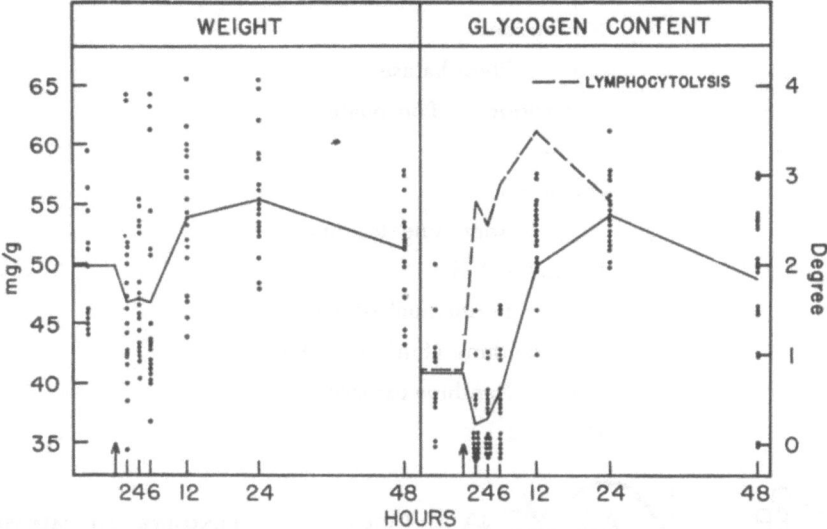

FIGURE 9. EFFECT OF 5–10MG/100G OF CORTISONE UPON LIVER OF RATS

tained in the pancreas. Its desoxyribose nucleic acid phosphorus content was found to be 181–261 mg per 100 gm of fresh tissue, a quantity which is much larger than that of any other tissue (60). It has often been demonstrated that the disintegrating lymphocytes are taken up by macrophages which rapidly digest their nucleoproteins.

The degradation of nucleic acids and some of the enzymes concerned with this degradation are given in Table 3. A study of the activity of adenosine deaminase and xanthine oxidase in lymphoid tissue was reported by Wagner and Ehrich (61). It was found that following the injection of a vaccine into the foot pad of rabbits the adenosinase activity rises with the activity of or lymphocytolysis in the germinal centers; it was not related to antibody formation or the concentration of desoxyribose or ribose nucleic acid in the nodes (Fig. 10). Xanthine oxidase activity, on the other hand, was not observed. As Dr. Wagner was inducted into the Army, we could not continue this work, but it was suggested that the significance of lymphocytolysis may lie in the delivery

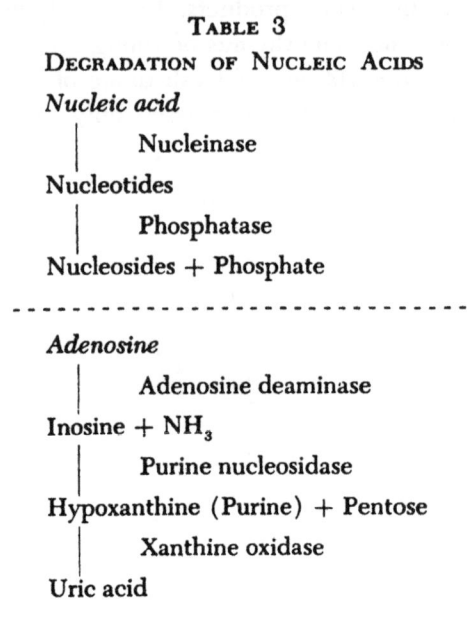

TABLE 3
DEGRADATION OF NUCLEIC ACIDS

Nucleic acid
　　| Nucleinase
Nucleotides
　　| Phosphatase
Nucleosides + Phosphate

- -

Adenosine
　　| Adenosine deaminase
Inosine + NH$_3$
　　| Purine nucleosidase
Hypoxanthine (Purine) + Pentose
　　| Xanthine oxidase
Uric acid

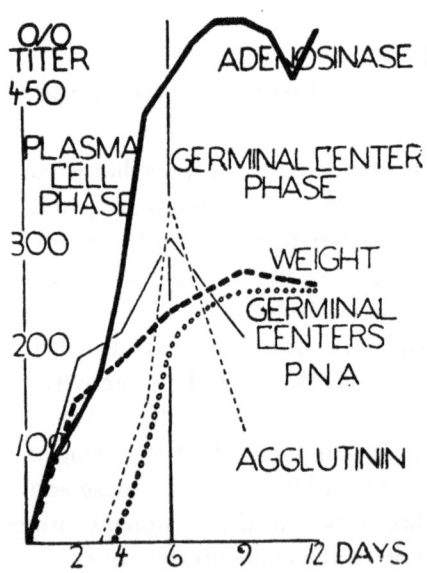

FIGURE 10. ADENOSINE DEAMINASE ACTIVITY COMPARED WITH THE ACTIVITY OF OR LYMPHOCYTOLYSIS IN THE GERMINAL CENTERS AND WITH THE CONCENTRATION OF RIBOSE NUCLEIC ACID (PNA) AND ANTIBODY IN THE POPLITEAL LYMPH NODES OF RABBITS FOLLOWING A SINGLE INJECTION OF A VACCINE INTO THE FOOT PAD Note that the curve of adenosine deaminase activity resembles that of the germinal centers, while PNA and antibody concentration reached their peak on the 6th day and then declined sharply.

of purines and pyrimidines and other split products of nucleoproteins. As purines have been shown to be powerful stimuli of phosphorylation, or, more precisely, they act as phosphorus transferring enzymes (Polis and others) (62), our results may be interpreted to mean that lymphocytolysis furnishes not only building stones but also energy for synthetic processes. If this were true, we would understand why lymphocytes are formed continually, why they are dispersed throughout the body, and why they are removed after a life span of possibly less than a day. We should comprehend also why lymphocytolysis is associated with or preceded by swelling of reticuloendothelial cells; these are the cells which contain the enzymes necessary for the degradation of nucleic acids.

However this may be, we feel that lymphocytolysis plays a basic role not only in the action of steroid hormones but also in physiology in general. We also believe that it furnishes a clue to the function of the lymphocyte.

Summary.—Corticosteroids have a depressing effect upon lymphoid tissue. The 11-oxy- and hydroxycorticosteroids are more effective than the sex hormones, while the desoxycorticosteroids depress lymphoid tissue only in large doses. The augmentation of this effect by stress and the ineffectiveness of the steroids upon washed-cell suspensions suggest that they require cofactors for their action.

Lymphocytolysis is a normal function of germinal centers. Pathological lymphocytolysis is seen best in the cortex of the thymus, plasmocytolysis in the medullary cords of lymph nodes. Grading of the degree of these phenomena reveals two phases. The second of these is suppressed by dibenamine; the first is not. While lymphocytolysis is associated with increased phagocytosis by macrophages, no conspicuous ingestion of disintegrating plasma cells was observed. Lymphocytolysis and plasmocytolysis furnish protein and nucleic acids and their split products. Protein may be used for gluconeogenesis, while nucleic acids and their split products may furnish building stones and energy for synthesis in general.

REFERENCES

1. Selye, H., Thymus and adrenals in the response of the organism to injuries and intoxications, *Brit. J. Exp. Path.*, 1936, 17:234.
2. Paltauff, A., Ueber die Beziehungen der Thymus zum plötzlichen Tod,

Wien. klin. Woschr., 1889, 2:877; 1890, 3:172; *Berl. klin. Woschr.* 1892, 29:298.
3. Jaffe, H. L., The influence of the suprarenal gland on the thymus; I: Regeneration of the thymus following double suprarenalectomy in the rat; II: Direct evidence of regeneration of the involved thymus following double suprarenalectomy in the rat; III: Stimulation of the growth of the thymus gland following double suprarenalectomy in young rats, *J. Exp. Med.*, 1924, 40:325, 619, 753.
4. Marine, D., Status lymphaticus, *Arch. Path.*, 1928, 5:661.
5. Marine, D., O. T. Mauley, and E. J. Baumann, The influence of thyroidectomy, gonadectomy, suprarenalectomy, and splenectomy on the thymus gland of rabbits, *J. Exp. Med.*, 1924, 40:429.
6. Selye, H., Studies on adaptation, *Endocrinology*, 1937, 21:169.
7. ——— The general adaptation syndrome and the diseases of adaptation, *J. Clin. Endocrinology*, 1946, 6:117.
8. ——— Stress, Acta Inc., Montreal, 1950.
9. ——— Thymus, adrenals and thyroid in the response of the organism to certain drugs, *Am. J. Physiol.*, 1936, 116:141.
10. Selye, H., C. M. Harlow, and J. B. Collip, Über die Auslösung der Alarmreaktion mit Follikelhormon, *Endokrinologie*, 1936, 18:81.
11. Carriere, G., G. Morel, and P. J. Gineste, Influence de l'adrenaline et de l'extrait cortico-surrenal sur le thymus du lapin et du rat, *C. R. Soc. Biol.*, 1937, 126:46.
12. Ingle, D. J., Atrophy of the thymus in normal and hypophysectomized rats following administration of cortin, *Proc. Soc. Exp. Biol. & Med.*, 1938, 38:443.
13. Ingle, D. J., G. M. Higgins, and E. C. Kendall, Atrophy of the adrenal cortex in the rat produced by administration of large amounts of cortin, *Anat. Rec.*, 1938, 71:363.
14. Ingle, D. J., and H. L. Mason, Subcutaneous administration of cortin compounds in solid form to the rat, *Proc. Soc. Exp. Biol. & Med.*, 1938, 39:154.
15. Wells, B. B., and E. C. Kendall, A qualitative difference in the effect of compounds separated from the adrenal cortex on distribution of electrolytes and on atrophy of the adrenals and thymus glands of rats, *Proc. Staff Meet. Mayo Clin.*, 1940, 15:133, 324.
16. Dougherty, T. F., and A. White, Influence of hormones on lymphoid tissue structure and function; the role of the pituitary adrenotropic hormone in the regulation of the lymphocytes and other cellular elements of the blood, *Endocrinology*, 1944, 35:1.
17. ——— Functional alterations in lymphoid tissue induced by adrenal cortical secretion, *Am. J. Anat.*, 1945, 77:81.
18. ——— An evaluation of alterations produced in lymphoid tissue by pituitary-adrenal cortical secretion, *J. Lab. & Clin. Med.*, 1947, 32:584.

19. Selye, H., Interactions between various steroid hormones, *Can. M.A.J.*, 1940, 42:113.
20. —— Variations in organ size caused by chronic treatment with adrenal cortical compounds, *J. Anat.*, 1941/2, 76:94.
21. Selye, H., and S. Albert, The effect of various steroids in intact male rats, *Am. J. Med. Sc.*, 1942, 204:876.
22. Selye, H., and C. E. Hall, Pathological changes induced in various species by overdosage with desoxycorticosterone, *Arch. Path.*, 1943, 36:19.
23. Ingle, D. J., Effect of two steroid compounds on weight of thymus of adrenalectomized rats, *Proc. Soc. Exp. Biol. & Med.*, 1940, 44:174.
24. Dontigny, P., The morphological effect of desoxycorticosterone acetate on the thymus, *Proc. Soc. Exp. Biol. & Med.*, 1946, 63:248.
25. Carnes, W. H., C. Ragan, J. W. Ferrebee, and J. O'Neill, Effects of desoxycorticosterone acetate in the albino rat, *Endocrinology*, 1941, 29:144.
26. Moon, H. D., Inhibition of somatic growth in castrate rats with pituitary extracts, *Proc. Soc. Exp. Biol. & Med.*, 1936, 37:34.
27. Simpson, M. E., and others, Similarity of response of thymus and lymph nodes to administration of adrenocorticotropic hormone in the rat, *Proc. Soc. Exp. Biol. & Med.*, 1943, 54:135.
28. Cramer, W., and E. S. Horning, Hormonal relationship between the ovary and the adrenal gland and its significance in the etiology of mammary cancer, *Lancet*, 1939, 1:192.
29. Schacher, J., J. S. L. Browne, and H. Selye, Effect of various sterols on thymus in the adrenalectomized rat, *Proc. Soc. Exp. Biol. & Med.*, 1937, 36:488.
30. Selye, H., Effect of dosage on the morphogenetic actions of testosterone, *Proc. Soc. Exp. Biol. & Med.*, 1941, 46:142.
31. Selye, H., and G. Masson, The effect of estrogens as modified by adrenal insufficiency, *Endocrinology*, 1939, 25:211.
32. Selye, H., J. S. L. Browne, and J. B. Collip, Effect of large doses of progesterone in the female rat, *Proc. Soc. Exp. Biol. & Med.*, 1936, 34:472.
33. Evans, H. M., H. D. Moon, M. E. Simpson, and W. R. Lyons, Atrophy of thymus of the rat resulting from administration of adrenocorticotropic hormone, *Proc. Soc. Exp. Biol. & Med.*, 1938, 38:419.
34. Baker, B. L., D. J. Ingle, and C. H. Li, The histology of lymphoid organs of rats treated with adrenocorticotropin, *Am. J. Anat.*, 1951, 88:313.
35. Yoffey, J. M., and J. S. Baxter, Some effects of pituitary adrenotropic hormone (PATH), extract of suprarenal cortex, and colchicine on the haemopoietic system, *J. Anat.*, 1946, 80:132.
36. Robertson, J. S., Failure of adrenal cortical extracts to cause lysis of living lymphocytes in vitro, *Nature*, 1948, 161:814.
37. Dougherty, T. F., and A. White, Increased "plasma cell" production following adrenal cortical stimulation, *Anat. Rec.*, 1946, (Suppl.), 94:13.

38. Ehrich, W. E., J. Seifter, and G. M. Hudyma, Effect of the alarm reaction upon lymphocytes and plasma cells, *Fed. Proc.*, 1951, 10:354.
39. Reinhardt, W. O., and C. H. Li, Depression of lymphocyte content of thoracic duct lymph by adrenocorticotrophic hormone, *Science*, 1945, 101:360.
40. Yoffey, J. M., M. Reiss, and J. S. Baxter, Pituitary adrenotropic hormone, extract of suprarenal cortex, lymph, and lymphoid tissue, *Nature*, 1946, 157:368.
41. Dougherty, T. F. and A. White, Effect of pituitary adrenotropic hormone on lymphoid tissue, *Proc. Soc. Exp. Biol. & Med.*, 1943, 53:132.
42. Reinhardt, W. O., H. Aron, and C. H. Li, Effect of adrenocorticotrophic hormone on leucocyte picture of normal rats and dogs, *Proc. Soc. Exp. Biol. & Med.*, 1944, 57:19.
43. Delaunay, A., M. Delaunay, and J. Lebrun, Lésions et réactions du tissu lymphoide, *Ann. Inst. Pasteur*, 1949, 76:203.
44. Reiss, E., E. Mertens, and W. E. Ehrich, Agglutination of bacteria by lymphoid cells in vitro, *Proc. Soc. Exp. Biol. & Med.*, 1950, 74:732.
45. Schreck, R., Cytotoxic action of hormones of the adrenal cortex according to the method of unstained cell counts, *Endocrinology*, 1949, 45:317.
46. —— Color test to measure the toxicity of adrenal cortex hormones to lymphocytes, *Proc. Soc. Exp. Biol. & Med.*, 1951, 76:557.
47. Feldman, J. D., The in vitro reaction of cells to adrenal cortical steroids with special reference to lymphocytes, *Endocrinology*, 1950, 46:552.
48. Heilman, D. H., The effect of 11-dehydro-17-hydroxycorticosterone and 11-dehydrocorticosterone on lymphocytes in tissue culture, *Proc. Staff Meet. Mayo Clin.*, 1945, 20:310, 318.
49. Hechter, O., and S. Johnson, In vitro effect of adrenal cortical extract upon lymphocytolysis, *Endocrinology*, 1949, 45:351.
50. Herlant, M., Conditioning through stress of the action of corticosteroids on lymphoid organs, *Proc. Soc. Exp. Biol. & Med.*, 1950, 73:399.
51. Ehrich, W. E., and J. Seifter, Role played by the salivary glands in the "alarm reaction," *Arch. Path.*, 1948, 45:239.
52. Seifter, J., and W. E. Ehrich, Goitrogenic compounds: pharmacological and pathological effects, *J. Pharm. & Exp. Ther.*, 1948, 92:303.
53. Long, C. N. H., The conditions associated with the secretion of the adrenal cortex, *Fed. Proc.*, 1947, 6:461.
54. Seifter, J., W. E. Ehrich, A. J. Begany, and G. M. Hudyma, Epinephrine and dibenamine in the alarm reaction, *Fed. Proc.*, 1949, 8:331.
55. Ehrich, W. E., Cellular Sources of Antibodies, in Blood Cells and Plasma Proteins; Their State in Nature. New York, The Academic Press, 1953.
56. —— The role of the lymphocyte in the circulation of the lymph, *Ann. N. Y. Acad. Sci.*, 1946, 46:823.
57. Bergner, G. E., and H. W. Deane, Effects of pituitary adrenocorticotrophic hormone on the intact rat, with special reference to cytochemical changes in the adrenal cortex, *Endocrinology*, 1948, 43:240.

58. Dougherty, T. F., A. White, and J. H. Chase, Relationship of the effects of adrenal cortical secretion on lymphoid tissue and on antibody titer, *Proc. Soc. Exp. Biol. & Med.*, 1944, 56:28.
59. White, A., and T. F. Dougherty, Influence of pituitary adrenotrophic hormone on lymphoid tissue structure in relation to serum proteins, *Proc. Soc. Exp. Biol. & Med.*, 1944, 56:26.
60. Davidson, J. N., Some factors influencing the nucleic acid content of cells and tissues, *Cold Spring Harbor Symposium on Quantitative Biology*, 1947, 12:50.
61. Wagner, B., and W. E. Ehrich, Adenosinase, adenase and xanthine oxidase of lymphoid tissues, *Fed. Proc.*, 1950, 9:347.
62. Polis, B. D., E. Polis, and L. Jedeikin, The stimulating effect of xanthines on the aerobic formation of high energy phosphate, *Am. J. Med. Sc.*, 1950, 219:583.

Chapter 5

THE EFFECT OF CORTISONE UPON REPAIR PROCESSES IN DENSE AND LOOSE CONNECTIVE TISSUE [1]

By CHARLES RAGAN, RAFFAEL LATTES, J. W. BLUNT, JR., DE GUISE VAILLANCOURT, RALPH A. JESSAR, AND WALLACE EPSTEIN, *Departments of Medicine and Surgery and the Laboratory for Histochemistry of the Department of Orthopedic Surgery, Columbia University College of Physicians and Surgeons, and the Edward Daniels Faulkner Arthritis Clinic of the Presbyterian Hospital, New York*

CERTAIN GENERAL CONCEPTS concerning repair processes in connective tissue should be formulated before we attempt to discuss the modification of such processes by a specific agent. The first concept concerns the unsettled controvery surrounding the stem cell of the fibroblast in adult tissue. Although some of the evidence favors the hypothesis advanced by Maximov and Bloom (1) that fibroblasts are derived from mononuclear cells—call them macrophages if you will; for this discussion we will refer to the stem cell as the precursor of the fibroblast. The second concept is that inflammation and repair are intimately related and that one can scarcely be considered without including the other. Thus, if an inflammatory process is localized, obviously repair is taking place, and the earlier stages of repair are characterized by a mild inflammatory reaction. In the third concept, which is speculative, one may regard repair as an acute phase of growth and maintenance of body structure, including in this concept the thought that cells which play an active role in repair may play a similar role in normal tissue replacement and turnover. Thus, it may be assumed that in repair one is studying the growth of tissue at a markedly accelerated rate, with augmentation of the cell population normally responsible for growth.

Among the earliest observations on the effects of the purified adrenal hormones, such as cortisone and compound F in the experimental ani-

---

[1] Aided in part by a grant from the Masonic Foundation for Medical Research and Human Welfare, and with funds supplied by the U.S.P.H.S.

mal, were those concerning a decrease in rate of growth (2, 3). If our hypothesis is correct, it would be expected that there would be a retardation of repair following the administration of a potent hormone, such as cortisone, and this has been proven to be the case (4). The techniques used in evaluating the repair process are much cruder than growth curves in a standard strain of animal. They depend on morphological details which are static, requiring repeated observations in order to achieve a dynamic aspect and lend themselves poorly, if at all, to quantitative evaluation. Probably because of this lack of precision, larger amounts of hormones are required to demonstrate an effect upon repair than with the more accurate method involving observations of growth rates in the intact animal. The study of repair has one slight advantage, that of speed, since results may be obtained within a week in small animals such as the mouse. It further provides a larger observable cell population in the traumatized area.

The effect of cortisone on repair processes is delay, a deceleration of the process. It is apparently dependent on several factors.

1. *The amount of hormone injected.*—Roughly the lag in repair is related to the amount of hormone. With large doses, repair processes may be brought to a temporary standstill. With smaller doses, the tempo of the process is accelerated, until at a certain low level of hormone administration no appreciable modification may be found with our methods. At this level growth of the young animal may still be decreased. This is possibly a reflection of the crudeness of our technique.

2. *The nutrition of the animal.*—Findlay and Howes (5) have shown that a given dose of cortisone (ca 3 mgm/kg) in a fed rabbit delays the appearance of granulations while 1.5 mgm/kg does not. In a partially starved rabbit, however, repair is appreciably retarded at a dosage of 1.5 mgm/kg.

3. *The species of animal.*—We have established roughly the dosage relationships in several species of mammals, but our data are fairly extensive only for the rabbit and mouse. In a sick human being, with rheumatoid arthritis, lupus, and so forth, who is eating well, delay in repair is evident at a dosage of 2 to 3 mgm/kg. The rabbit at 3 mgm/kg, the adult dog at 10 mgm/kg, the guinea pig and rat at 50 mgm/kg, and the mouse at 75 to 100 mgm/kg demonstrate a similar retardation.

Deceleration of repair processes is apparent only when there is evidence of lymph node and thymic involution or when typical changes are observed in the spleen, all of which have been considered to be manifestations of the "hyperadrenal" state. Adrenal atrophy is not a necessary accompaniment, since delay in repair may be observed before atrophy has developed and also a similar delay in repair is seen following the administration of ACTH with resultant adrenal hypertrophy.

The effect of the hormone is local (6–9), since topical application gives findings similar to systemic administration. The change, as stated above, is solely a delay, since if an animal is wounded twice at intervals while cortisone is maintained, in the nine-day wound adequate healing is apparent, with possibly a somewhat decreased amount of scar tissue, whereas marked delay is seen in the five-day wound.

The process of repair may be separated into two distinct phases. In the first, cellular infiltration and edema are present and a change in the appearance of collagen may be seen, namely, tapering of the end of collagen fibers. In the second phase, macrophages are still present, and more new fibroblasts appear, with the usual elements of the scar. In our experiments the most dramatic effects of the hormone have been exerted in the second phase, while there is relatively little difference between the control and the cortisone-treated animal in the first phase. Frequently there appears to be little or no tapering of the collagen, and the cut fibers often retain their blunt appearance and there is less endothelial swelling in the cortisone-treated animal. This has been observed when using wounds, viruses, fractures, and foreign bodies as injuring agents. The duration of the first phase has varied with different stimuli. In general, it has lasted for twelve hours in vaccinia virus infection in rabbits and from one to two days in skin wounds and the foreign body reaction to cotton gauze in rabbits, rats, and mice. In the fracture experiments on rabbits (10) in which the fractures were not immobilized, the first phase, or latent period, has lasted four days. Possibly this longer period was due to persistent trauma induced by weight-bearing in the fractured extremity. Michael (11) has presented evidence to show that the effect of cortisone could be observed from the moment of initiation of the inflammatory stimulus. Using croton oil as the irritant, he has described fewer inflammatory cells, less edema, and less margination of leucocytes from the onset of the inflammatory reaction. In our studies, in the first phase, with large doses of hormone, we have seen no appreciable difference in edema and cellular infiltration in control and cortisone-treated animals (Figure 1). Whether the difference between Michael's observations and ours is qualitative or quantitative has not been established. In the second phase of the reaction, that is, within twenty-four hours following vaccinia virus infection, within two to three days after trauma of various kinds, and within five days in the fracturing experiments, the difference between control and cortisone-treated animals becomes manifest. In the cortisone-treated animal, in the second phase, there is a decrease in the components of the repair reactions, for example, edema, mononuclear cells (macrophages) fibroblasts, endothelial swelling, capillary buds and angioplasia, metachromatic material, and collagen (Figure 2). There is also less differentiation into specialized cells concerned with bone deposition, leading to less cartilage and osteoid and fewer chondrocytes. There is, as well, less reaction to cotton gauze with fewer macrophages and no foreign-body giant cells.

The cellular effect appears to be exerted on the precursor of the fibroblast, since once fibroblasts and new blood vessels have appeared, repair follows. Regardless of the controversy concerning the origin of the fibroblast, the chain of events starts at the capillary. One theory postulates that cells migrate through the wall, become macrophages, and thence fibroblasts. The other school feels that the stem cell of the fibroblast derives from undifferentiated mesenchymal cells located in the vicinity of blood vessels. In either event, cells which are absent from an area before trauma appear following trauma, thus implying migration or proliferation.

Because of the scarcity of macrophages seen in a traumatized area in the second phase of repair following cortisone administration, several possibilities have required exploration. Consequently, the capacity of the macrophage to reach an area and to migrate into an area and its ability to phagocytize have been investigated. Schmidt and Squires (12), following the theories of Maximow (13), feel that there are smaller numbers of macrophages available to the area because of the restraining effect of the hormone on lymphocyte production through suppression of lymph node metabolism. In tissue culture (14), although migration of lymphocytes was decreased by cortisone, migration of macrophages was not affected. Phagocytic activity of macrophages in the liver (15) and in the spleen (16) is apparently unaffected by the administration of the adrenal hormones.

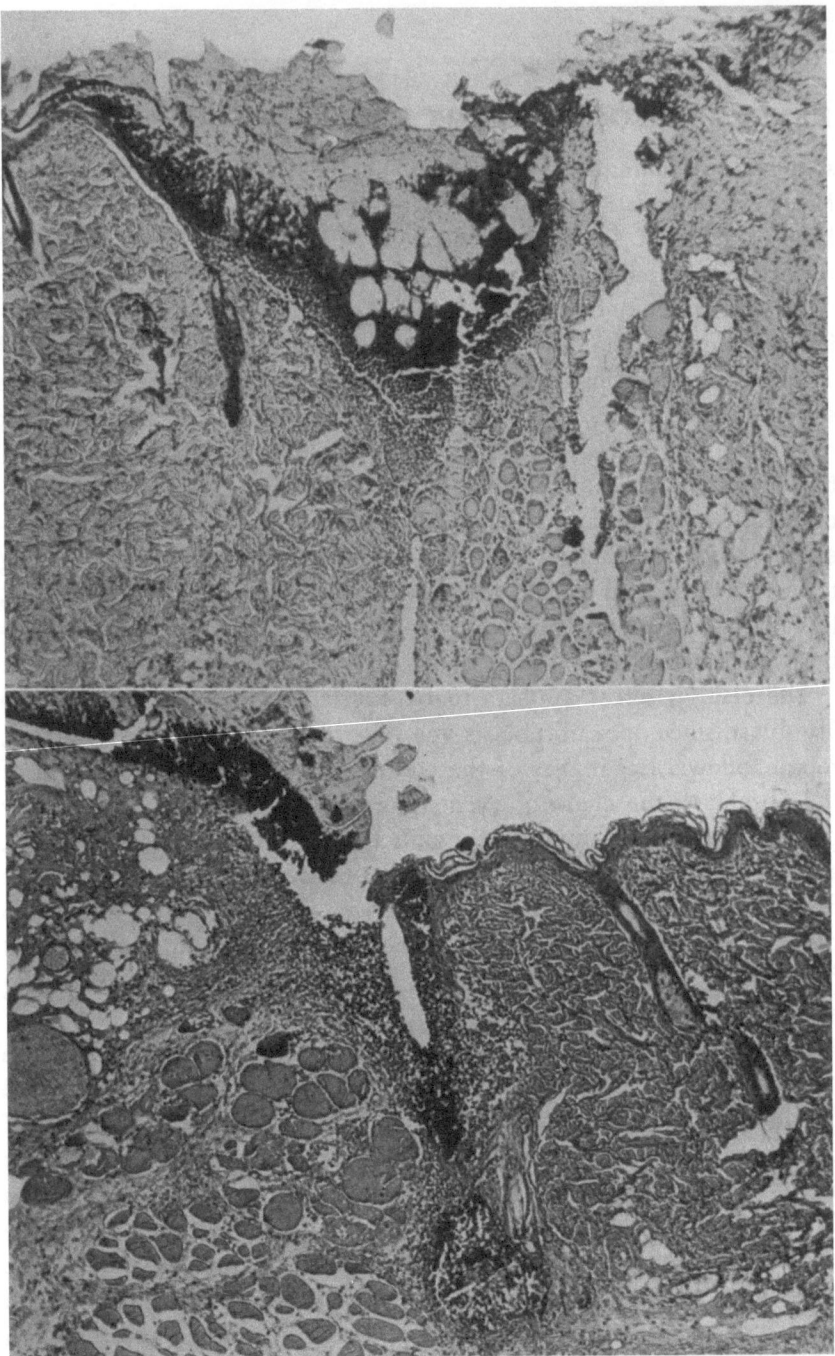

FIGURE 1. TWENTY-FOUR-HOUR SKIN WOUND

Above. Rat 13C, Control; twenty-four-hour skin wound, the dermis and underlying layers showing polymorphonuclear leucocytic infiltration and moderate edema (H & E, ×97)

Below. Rat 14E, Cortisone-treated; twenty-four-hour skin wound, showing a zone of polymorphonuclear leucocytic infiltration in the dermis on both sides of the recent incision and moderate edema of the dense collagenous tissue (H & E, ×97)

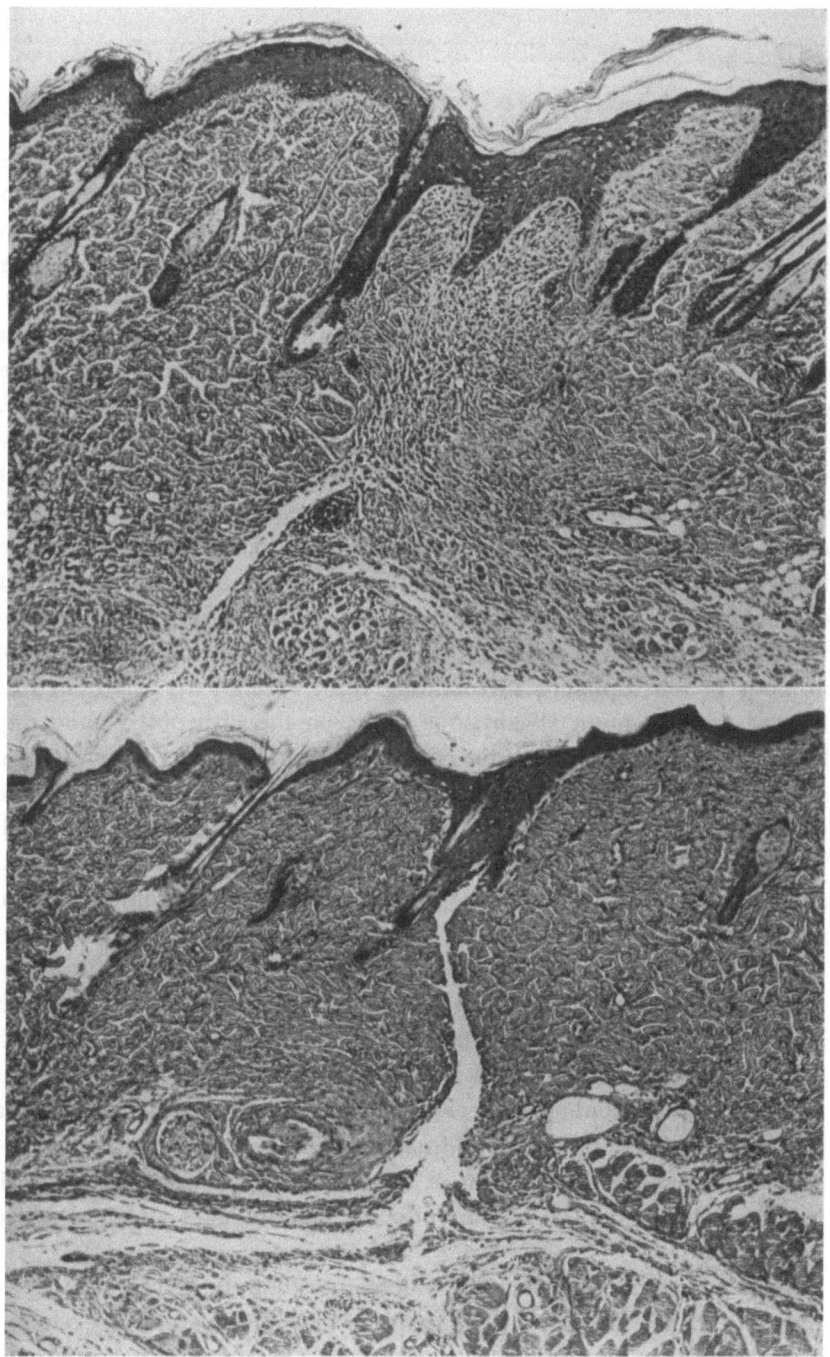

FIGURE 2. FIVE-DAY SKIN WOUND

Above. Rat 21C, control; five-day skin wound, showing complete epithelial repair, the gap in the dermis being completely filled with young connective tissue (H & E, ×97)

Below. Rat 21E, cortisone-treated; five-day skin wound, showing regenerated epithelium over the gap in the dermis, which is still open and shows no signs of reaction to injury (H & E, ×97)

In the fascial and omental spreads of rats given trypan blue intramuscularly many macrophages containing trypan blue were seen throughout the spread in cortisone-treated animals, and although quantitation is difficult, it was our impression that there were more cells containing the dye in cortisone-treated animals than in the controls. Thus, although macrophages are scarce in an area of inflammation in a cortisone-treated animal, the inability of macrophages to migrate while under the influence of cortisone has not been apparent in tissue culture, and macrophages have retained their ability to phagocytize actively when foreign material was brought to them. Schmidt's (12) theory that a dearth of macrophages is caused by a decreased supply of their precursors as a result of cortisone treatment would still be tenable were it not for one observation we have made. We have inserted many types of foreign substances into subcutaneous tunnels (17) in cortisone-treated rats and have observed, as expected, a marked decrease in the number of macrophages surrounding these foreign materials. In rats treated with 10 mgm of cortisone daily, on the fifth post-wound day there has been relatively little reaction surrounding the cotton gauze, and in many instances the gauze lay free in the tunnel (Figure 3). To date, the introduction of only one substance has consistently been followed by a macrophage response on the fifth day in cortisone-treated rats, namely, oxidized gauze, a polymer of cellubiuronic acid. In cortisone-treated rats there has been a marked response to oxidized cellulose of cells resembling macrophages, a reaction similar in all respects to that seen in the control animal (Figure 4)—while skin wounds in the same animal have continued to show retardation of repair. It therefore seems possible that in the cortisone-treated animal there is no dearth of macrophage precursors. The absence of these cells from a traumatized area in cortisone-treated animals may result from the suppression of the elaboration of a substance which normally constitutes a stimulus for the accumulation of macrophages and new blood vessels.

Oxidized cellulose is an acid mucopolysaccharide, and at least two possibilities are raised: (1) the material may act as a cation exchange resin leading to an area of lowered pH, or (2) the material may have properties similar to the acid mucopolysaccharides present in normal and traumatized tissue. Both these possibilities are now being explored.

In conclusion, our evidence tends to indicate that the effect of cor-

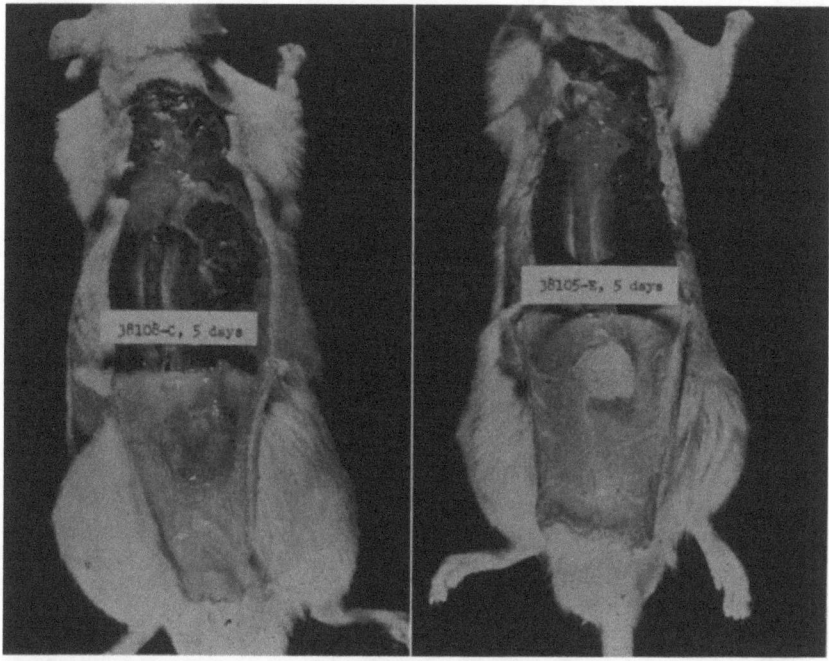

FIGURE 3. CONTROL RAT (38108-C) AND CORTISONE-TREATED RAT (38105-E) AUTOPSIED FIVE DAYS FOLLOWING SUBCUTANEOUS IMPLANTATION OF GAUZE PLEDGET
Note the complete encapsulation of the foreign body in the control animal and showing free gauze and unaffected surrounding tissues in the cortisone-treated animal

tisone on the repair process is exerted chiefly during the second phase of this process. In the first place the microscopic appearance is similar to that seen in the untreated animal, save, perhaps, for a lack of collagen degeneration and less endothelial swelling. It seems likely that in the second phase there is a decreased elaboration of a substance or substances having chemotactic or stimulating properties for macrophages, fibroblasts, and new blood vessels.

REFERENCES

1. Maximov, A. A., and W. Bloom, Textbook of Histology, W. B. Saunders Co., Philadelphia, Pa. 1948, Chapters IV–V.
2. Ingle, D. J., R. Sheppard, E. A. Aberle, and M. H. Kuizenga. A comparison of the acute effects of corticosterone and 17-hydroxycorticosterone on

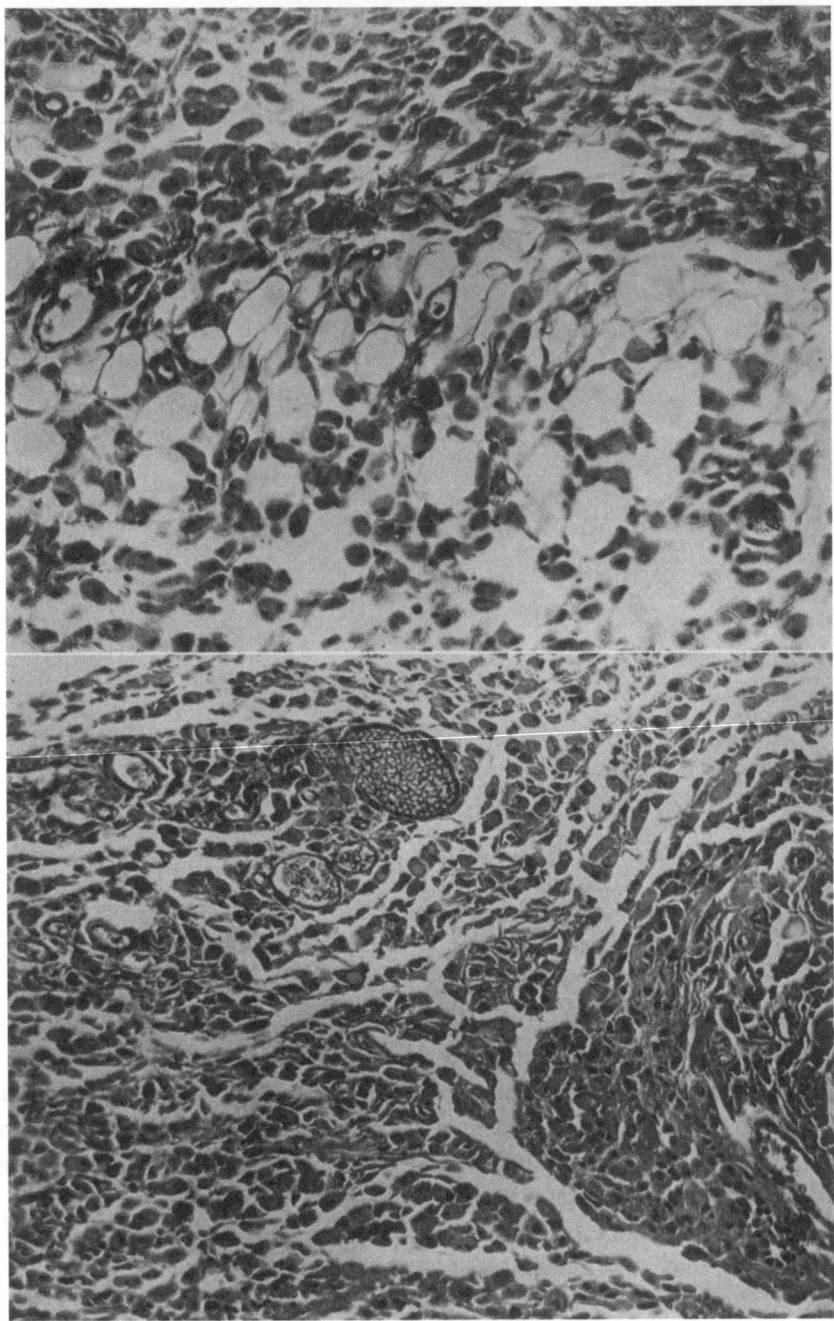

FIGURE 4. TISSUES OF TWO RATS SIX DAYS AFTER SUBCUTANEOUS IMPLANTATION OF OXYDIZED CELLULOSE

Above. Control rat (11CWO); note absence of any fibro or angioblastic proliferation and of inflammatory reaction, except for the large numbers of mononuclear cells of the histiocytic type, with basophilic cytoplasm (H & E, ×210).

Below. Cortisone-treated rat (10EWO): note enormous numbers of basophilic large mononuclears, of histiocytic type, and absence of inflammatory or fibroblastic reaction (H & E, ×210).

body weight and the urinary excretion of sodium chloride, potassium, nitrogen in the normal rat, *Endocrinology*, 1946, 39:52.
3. Wells, B. B., and E. C. Kendall, A qualitative difference in the effect of compounds separated from the adrenal cortex on distribution of electrolytes and on atrophy of the adrenal and thymus glands of rats, *Proc. Staff Meet. Mayo Clinic*, 1940, 15:133.
4. Ragan, C., E. L. Howes, C. M. Plotz, K. Meyer, J. W. Blunt, and R. Lattes, The effect of ACTH and cortisone on connective tissue, *Bull. N.Y. Acad. Med.*, 1950, 26:251.
5. Findlay, C. W., Jr., and E. L. Howes, The combined effect of cortisone and partial protein depletion on wound healing. *New England J. Med.*, 1952, 246:597.
6. Castor, C. W., and B. L. Baker, Local actions of adrenocortical steroids on epidermis and connective tissue of skin, *Endocrinology*, 1950, 47:234.
7. Howes, E. L., C. M. Plotz, J. W. Blunt, and C. Ragan. Retardation of wound healing by cortisone, *Surgery*, 1950, 28:177.
8. Jones, I. S., and K. Meyer, Inhibition of vascularization of the rabbit cornea by local application of cortisone, *Proc. Soc. Exp. Biol. & Med.*, 1950, 74:102.
9. Shapiro, R., B. Taylor, and M. Taubenhaus, Local effects of cortisone on granulation tissue and the role of denervation and ischemia, *Proc. Soc. Exp. Biol. & Med.*, 1951, 76:854.
10. Blunt, J. W., Jr., C. M. Plotz, R. Lattes, E. L. Howes, K. Meyer, and C. Ragan. The effect of cortisone on experimental fractures in the rabbit, *Proc. Soc. Exp. Biol. & Med.*, 1950, 73:678.
11. Michael, M., Jr., and C. M. Whorton, Delay of the early inflammatory response by cortisone, *Proc. Soc. Exp. Biol. & Med.*, 1951, 76:754.
12. Schmidt, L. H., and W. L. Squires, The influence of cortisone on primate malaria, *J. Exp. Med.*, 1951, 94:501.
13. Maximow, A. Cultures of blood leucocytes; from lymphocyte and monocyte to connective tissue, *Arch. f. exp. Zellforsch.*, 1928, 5:169.
14. Heilman, D. H. The effect of 11-dehydro-17-hydroxycorticosterone and 11-dehydrocorticosterone on the migration of macrophages in tissue culture, *Proc. Staff Meet. Mayo Clinic*, 1945, 20:318.
15. Lurie, M. B., P. Zappasodi, and A. M. Dannenberg, Jr. Effect of cortisone on the pathogenesis of tuberculosis, *Fed. Proc.*, 1951, 10:414.
16. Gordon, A. S., and G. Katsh, Relation of the adrenal cortex to the increased macrophagic activity induced by starvation, *Ann. N.Y. Acad. Sci.*, 1949, 52:1.
17. Lattes, R., and V. K. Frantz, Absorbable sponge tests, *Ann. Surg.*, 1945, 121:894.

Chapter 6

ADRENAL HORMONES AND THE DEVELOPMENT OF ANTIBODY AND HYPERSENSITIVITY [1]

By EDWARD E. FISCHEL, *The Department of Medicine, Columbia University College of Physicians and Surgeons and the Edward Daniels Faulkner Arthritis Clinic of the Presbyterian Hospital, New York*

IN THE TWO YEARS which have elapsed since our brief summary of studies on the relationship of adrenal cortical hormone to immune responses (1), there have appeared numerous reports devoted to this subject. It is not possible to review this work critically in the time available. Furthermore, in many instances the data are based on the study of heterogeneous systems and have not been strictly quantitative. Quantitative studies are necessary, since the development and severity of hypersensitivity depend largely on the quantity of antibody available for reaction in the tissues (2). There are, therefore, at least three questions to consider in connection with the study of immune responses; first, what is the effect of adrenal cortical hormones on the development of antibody; secondly, given a known amount of antibody, what effect does adrenal cortical hormone have on well-defined sensitivity reactions due to the union of antigen and antibody; finally, what effect do the hormones have on tissue reactivity nonspecifically rather than on the allergic reaction per se. Our discussion will be principally concerned with the first two questions and with the third only by implication.

In collaboration with Drs. Bjørneboe and Stoerk several series of rabbits were immunized to a polyvalent pneumococcus vaccine. A decided inhibition of antibody formation was found when cortisone or ACTH was administered during immunization (3). Table 1 illustrates the experiments with cortisone at two different dosage levels. It is apparent that there was considerable variation within all the groups, but at nine and fourteen days after onset of immunization the mean amount of

---

[1] Aided by grants from the Helen Hay Whitney Foundation and the Masonic Foundation for Medical Research and Human Welfare.

TABLE 1

The Effect of Cortisone on the Amount of Circulating Antibody When the Hormone Is Administered from the Onset of Immunization with Pneumococci

MG ANTIBODY NITROGEN PER ML OF SERUM (MG AbN/ML)

	10 MG CORTISONE I.M. DAILY		2.5 MG CORTISONE I.M. DAILY	
Rabbit	Ninth Day	Fourteenth Day	Rabbit	Fourteenth Day
B2	0.06	0.46	E24	0.49
B6	0.06	0.48	E8	0.62
B12	0.09		E29	0.67
B9	0.10	0.48	E20	0.70
B1	0.13		E28	0.80
B7	0.18	0.77	E26	0.85
			E23	0.85
			E5	0.85
			E27	1.06
			E7	1.19
Mean AbN/ml	0.12	0.55		0.81
Mean AbN/ml of control groups without cortisone	0.27 [a]	1.47 [a]		1.17 [b]

[a] 0.27 and 1.47 are the average AbN/ml on the 9th and 14th days, respectively, of 27 rabbits immunized simultaneously with the B group animals. Individual titers of these controls on the 9th and 14th days are as follows: 0.13, 0.49; 0.28, 0.54; 0.19, 0.60; 0.21, 0.61; 0.07, 0.69; 0.31, 0.75; 0.22, 0.99; 0.32, 1.12; 0.23, 1.15; 0.19, 1.20; 0.16, 1.26; 0.36, 1.33; 0.28, 1.34; 0.27, 1.54; 0.40, 1.54; 0.22, 1.57; 0.37, 1.61; 0.12, 1.68; 0.35, 1.68; 0.22, 1.95; 0.17, 2.16; 0.16, 2.23; 0.27, 2.34; 0.52, 2.40; 0.43, 2.52; 0.31, 3.05; 0.47 (9th day only).

[b] 1.17 is the average antibody nitrogen level per ml on the 14th day of 11 untreated control animals immunized simultaneously with the E group animals. These controls had the following titers: 0.41; 0.52; 0.71; 0.85; 1.04; 1.11; 1.19; 1.34; 1.46; 2.04; 2.18.

antibody nitrogen in rabbits given 10 mgm cortisone daily was about one half and one third, respectively, of the mean titer of untreated rabbits. At a dosage level of 2.5 mgm of cortisone daily there was less difference between treated and control groups. A distinct inhibition of antibody was also found with ACTH, even with the small dosage of ACTH used (Table 2).

In a previous study Bjørneboe and Gormsen (4) demonstrated a rough correlation of spleen weight with antibody titer in rabbits hyperimmunized by this method. A similar correlation was found in these studies.

TABLE 2

The Effect of ACTH on the Concentration of Circulating Antibody When the Hormone Is Administered from the Onset of Immunization with Pneumococci

MG ANTIBODY NITROGEN PER ML OF SERUM AT 14 AND AT 28 DAYS AFTER BEGINNING IMMUNIZATION WITH PNEUMOCOCCI

AFTER 14 DAYS		AFTER 28 DAYS	
ACTH Group P mg AbN/ml	Control Group K mg/AbN/ml	ACTH Group P mg/AbN/ml	Control Group K mg AbN/ml
0.50	0.98	0.67	1.41
0.54	1.47	1.01	1.90
0.62	1.49	1.22	2.30
0.81	2.02	1.67	...
2.34	2.22	3.34	5.31
	2.30		4.72
	2.50		6.23
Mean 0.96	1.85	1.58	3.65

Five New Zealand red rabbits treated with ACTH, approximately 0.5 to 1.0 mg Armour standard, every 8 hours for the entire period; 7 control rabbits of same strain.

The spleen of the cortisone-treated animals was smaller, and its microscopic architecture was disrupted. The disturbance by cortisone was found to involve numerous cell types of the spleen and lymph nodes (3).

It was of interest to observe what happens when cortisone is administered after immunization has already become well established. After fourteen days of immunization animals with varying levels of antibody were separated into two groups, one of which then was treated with cortisone. The immunizing injections of pneumococci were continued in both groups. Figure 1 illustrates the progressive increase in the mean titer of the control group of rabbits and the lack of any increase in the mean titer of the cortisone-treated group. There were widespread individual variations in both groups, but the pattern induced by cortisone was well defined. Another series of rabbits was treated with cortisone after immunization was well established, with similar results (Fig. 2). Continuation of cortisone for a longer period of time resulted in a distinct drop in antibody titer, despite the persistent administration of pneumococcus vaccine.

Antibody depression by cortisone or ACTH both during immunization and after the onset of immunization had not been observed by

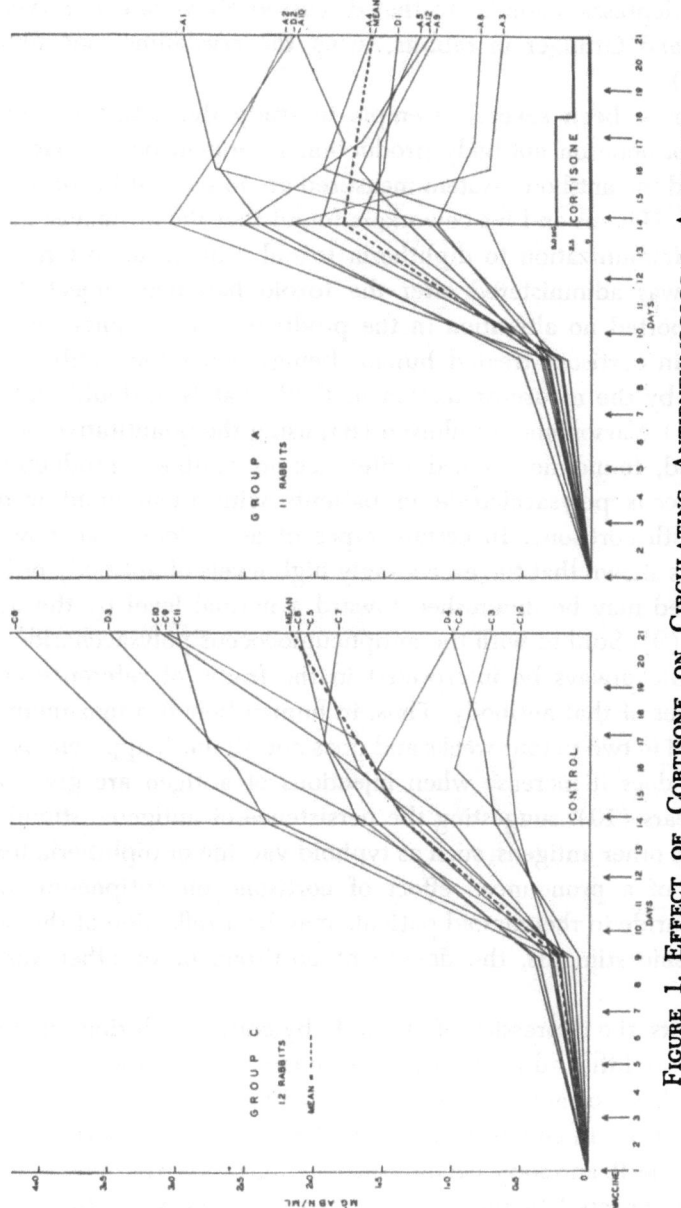

FIGURE 1. EFFECT OF CORTISONE ON CIRCULATING ANTIPNEUMOCOCCAL ANTIBODY NITROGEN PER ML SERUM (AB N/ML)
From J. Exp. Med., 1951, 93:37.

previous investigators in this field, as has been discussed elsewhere (3, 42). However, when quantitative immunochemical methods were employed, a depression similar to that discussed above was observed by Germuth and Ottinger in rabbits, using the crystalline egg albumin system (5).

There have been several attempts to study the action of adrenal cortical hormone on antibody production in human beings. Hormone dosage and the antibody system measured are important in considering the results. Havens and his coworkers found that the hormones had no effect on immunization to diphtheria toxoid, but in all instances the hormone was administered after the toxoid had been injected (6). Mirick reported no alteration in the production of antipneumococcus antibody in cortisone-treated human beings when the antibody was measured by the mouse-protection method, that is, a double dilution technic (7). Larson and Tomlinson (8), using the quantitative precipitin method, found no marked difference in antibody production to pneumococcus polysaccharide in patients with rheumatoid arthritis treated with cortisone. In certain types of acute leukemia, however, Larson has shown that the exceedingly high levels of antibody ordinarily obtained may be diminished toward a normal level by the use of cortisone (9). Studies with the antipneumococcus polysaccharide antibody should always be interpreted in the frame of reference of the peculiarities of that antibody. Thus, in human beings a maximum titer is achieved in two to four weeks and does not diminish appreciably with time, nor does it increase when injections of antigen are given after several years (10), suggesting the persistence of antigenic stimulus in contrast to other antigens, such as typhoid vaccine or diphtheria toxoid. The lack of a pronounced effect of cortisone on antipneumococcus polysaccharide in rheumatoid patients may be a reflection of the peculiar antigenic stimulus, the dosage of cortisone or of other variable factors.

In rabbits, the depression of antibody by cortisone during immunization suggested that adrenal cortical hormone acts by either accelerating the breakdown of antibody or inhibiting its synthesis. An experiment was carried out in collaboration with Drs. Stoerk and Bjørneboe (11) to determine if antibody catabolism was affected. Antibody was passively administered to four rabbits, two of which were treated with cortisone before and during passive immunization. The residual anti-

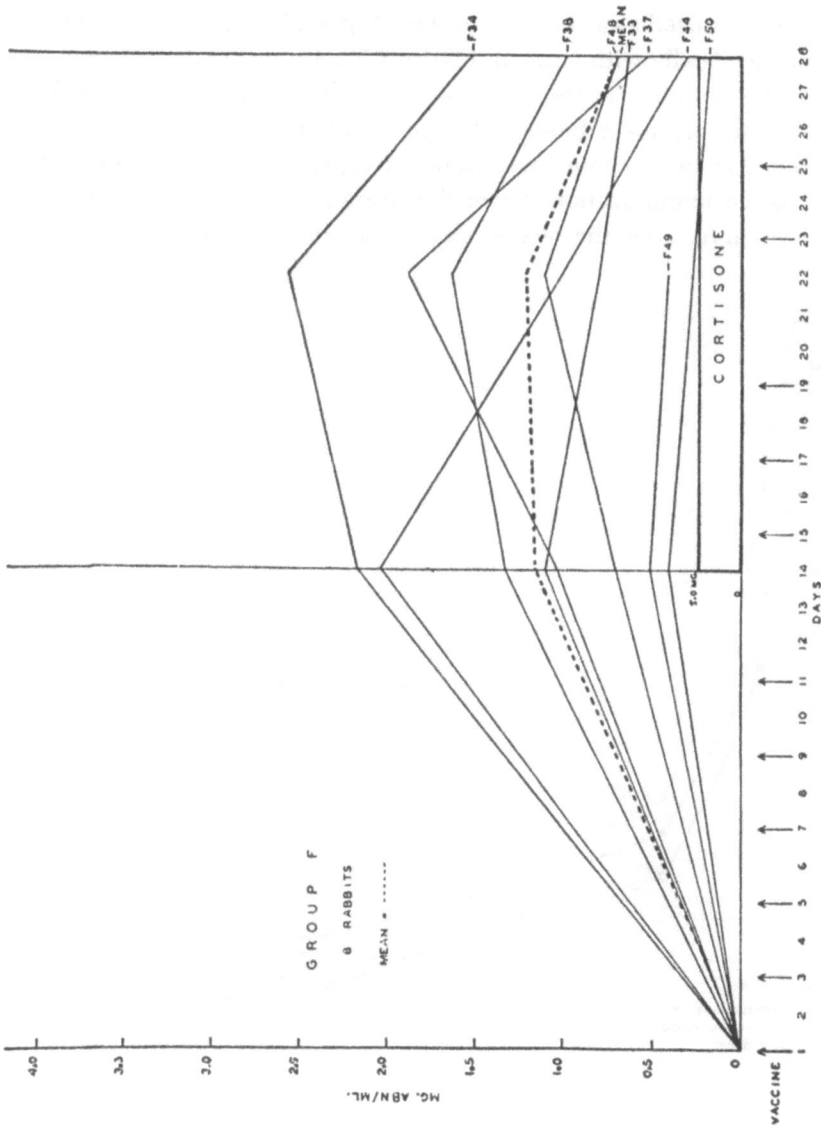

FIGURE 2. EFFECT OF CORTISONE ON CIRCULATING ANTIPNEUMOCOCCAL ANTIBODY NITROGEN PER ML SERUM (AB N/ML)
From J. Exp. Med., 1951, 93:37

body in the rabbit circulation was determined by the quantitative agglutination method of Heidelberger and Kabat (12). The antibody, therefore, was used as a "tagged" protein, tagged by virtue of its ability to react specifically with antigen. Figure 3 illustrates the disappearance rates of this antibody in the four animals studied. The similarity of the curves is striking for a biological experiment. Residual antibody was determined at twenty minutes, and one, two, four, seven, and ten days after passive immunization. From the straight-line part of this disappearance curve, after the second day a maximum half-life of the pas-

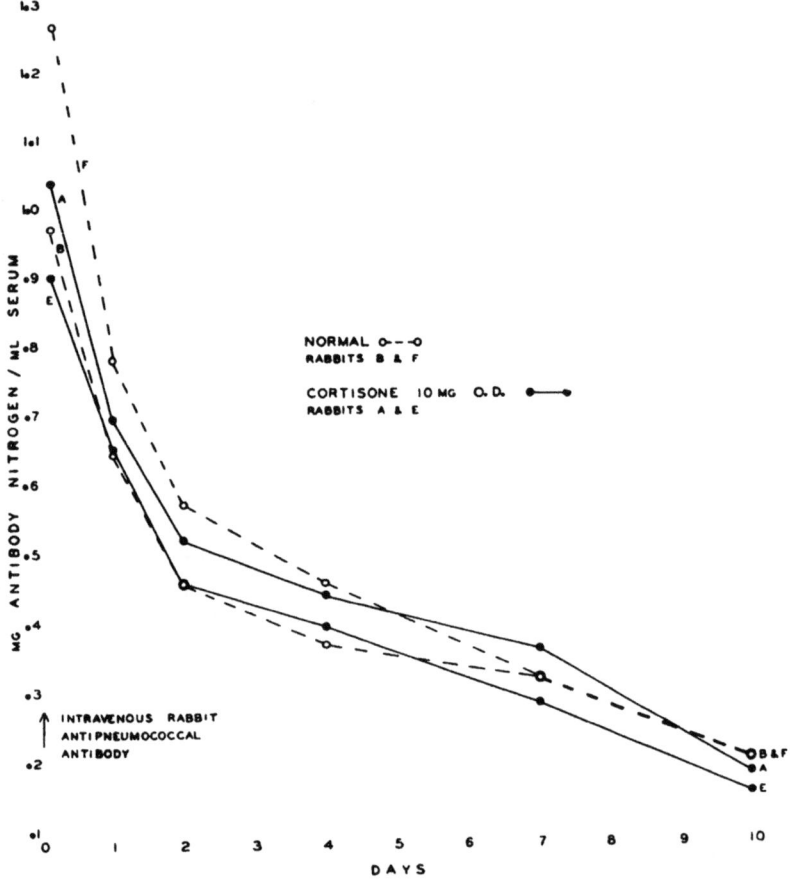

FIGURE 3. DISAPPEARANCE OF PASSIVELY ADMINISTERED ANTIBODY GLOBULIN FROM NORMAL AND CORTISONE-TREATED RABBITS
From Proc. Soc. Exp. Biol. & Med., 1951, 77:111.

sively administered antibody globulin is found to be about six days. This study demonstrated that antibody is not catabolized more rapidly in cortisone-treated animals and suggested rather that the cause of low antibody levels in immunized animals treated with hormone is inhibition of synthesis (11). This hypothesis is also supported by studies which show that labeled amino acids are not incorporated into tissue protein when cortisone is administered (13). Catabolism may be accelerated in other tisues, as mentioned by Dr. Engel (14), but for the antibody protein studied, at least, there was no indication of this. In order to test by immunochemical methods whether synthesis is inhibited, we have cast about for a situation in which protein is being synthesized at a very rapid rate, so rapid that degradation of the protein may be considered negligible in the early phase. Such a situation is found in the specific anamnestic, or secondary, response. If an animal has been immunized with a specific antigen and is then allowed to rest, the subsequent exposure to that antigen usually causes a marked increase in antibody. Within about 5 days large amounts of antibody may appear, in contrast to the slow and gradual increases which occur on initial immunization.

There is no substantial evidence that nonspecific stimuli can cause an outpouring of specific antibody. Eisen and his coworkers showed that adrenal extract failed to enhance circulating antibody (15). In 1949 our work with Drs. LeMay and Kabat showed that ACTH does not cause a nonspecific anamestic response, but, indeed, possibly even a diminution in antibody (16). DeVries has obtained similar quantitative immunochemical data (17), and other reports have now appeared confirming this finding, which is at variance with the findings of Dougherty and White (18).

In connection with the problem of inhibition of antibody synthesis by cortisone, we have returned to the study of anamnestic response, this time using crystalline egg albumin as the specific antigen to which the animals had previously been immunized. Precipitin reactions showed production of antibody protein was markedly inhibited in animals pretreated with cortisone. The rapid production of the globulin which occurs in untreated animals is absent in cortisone-treated animals (19; Fig. 4). A similar inhibition of the secondary response was reported by Stoerk in acute pyridoxine deficiency (20), and by Philips and others with nitrogen mustard. Fagraeus has obtained similar data on the inhibition of the secondary response, which is of great interest because of the time-dosage relationship (21). Fagraeus and Berglund gave rabbits an antigenic stimulus for a secondary response to typhoid bacilli and then, at various intervals, transplanted the spleens of these rabbits into recipient rabbits, some of which were treated with cortisone. Transplantation of the spleens of the donor rabbits was performed

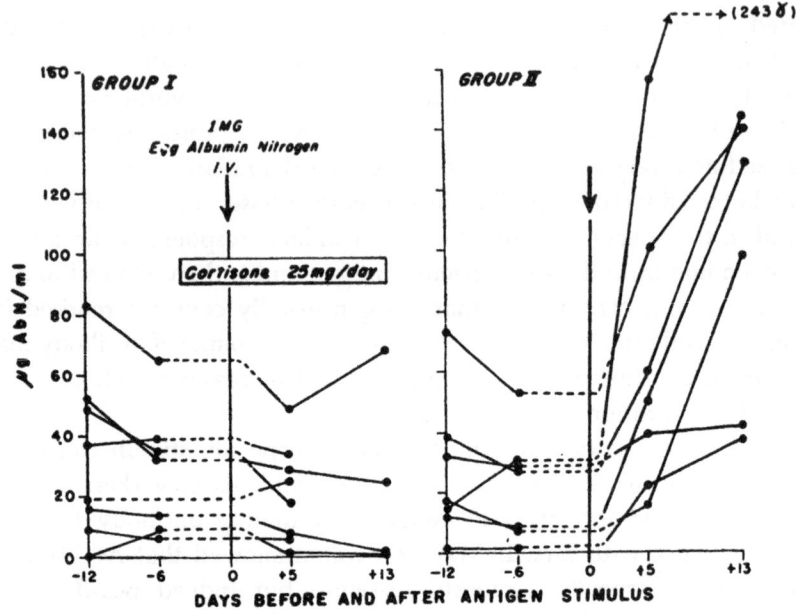

FIGURE 4. THE EFFECT OF CORTISONE ON ANTIBODY LEVELS OF RABBITS BEFORE AND AFTER THE INDUCTION OF A SECONDARY RESPONSE
From Proc. Soc. Exp. Biol. & Med., 1952, 81:344.

on either the first, second, or third day after antigen injection, but irrespective of the time of transplantation the recipient rabbits not treated with cortisone showed a great increase in titer of antibody to typhoid bacilli on the fourth or fifth day after the antigen was administered to the donor rabbit. In cortisone-treated recipient rabbits, transplantation during the first two days did not result in any antibody increase. When the spleen was transplanted three days after antigen was administered, the serum of the cortisone-treated recipient animal showed a rise in antibody on the fourth or fifth day similar to that of the control animal. It was concluded that cortisone did not inhibit the synthesis of antibody protein, but rather blocked the processes associated with assimilation of the antigen. Moeschlin and others have also reported that pretreatment with ACTH or cortisone inhibited the secondary response, while later treatment failed to do so, suggesting a similar effect caused by hormone administration (22). In studies on the inhibition by cortisone of experimentally induced acute disseminated encephalomyelitis in monkeys, Kabat, Wolf, and Bezer found that granuloma formation surrounding the site of antigen-adjuvant inoculation was reduced or abolished in the cortisone-treated animals (23). It had previously been shown that the granuloma formation was essential for the production of disseminated encephalomyelitis, presumably by bringing antibody forming cells in intimate association with the antigen (24). It would appear, from the studies on the lack of incorporation of isotopic amino acids into tissue proteins of cortisone-treated animals (13) and from the above studies, that both steps in the development of antibody may be affected by cortisone, that is, the "assimilation" of antigen and the synthesis of antibody globulin.

Having considered the effect of adrenal cortical hormone on antibody production as one of the aspects of the development of the immune response, the next logical consideration is the effect of hormone on well-defined sensitivity reactions due to the union of antigen and antibody. Anaphylaxis and the Arthus reaction, prototypes of allergic reactions, have been appraised quantitatively and found to exhibit a direct relationship between the amount of antibody available and the severity of reaction (2). It is to be expected, therefore, that those sensitivity reactions which are induced by active immunization may be inhibited to some extent by cortisone, since antibody production itself is inhibited. Studies on actively induced serum sickness (25) and the Arthus reaction (5) bear this out. By passive induction of the Arthus reaction, however, the effect of cortisone on antibody available for reaction is circumvented. It has been our experience that Arthus reactions induced by amounts of antibody resulting in minimal or maximal reactions are not altered by appreciable dosages of ACTH or cortisone (1). The failure of cortisone to affect the passive Arthus reactions has been corroborated by Germuth and Ottinger (5). On the other hand, it has been reported that passively induced systemic serum sickness reactions in rabbits have been inhibited by cortisone (26). This study may indicate a variable effect of cortisone in sites other than the skin, although it appears difficult to evaluate effects with precision in a system which results in numerous and widespread histological lesions.

It was early reported that anaphylaxis to horse serum in guinea pigs was not apparently altered by ACTH (27). Our own studies, employing known amounts of antibody to induce anaphylaxis according to the method of Kabat and his coworkers (2), confirmed the lack of effect of cortisone and of ACTH (1). Recently, with Dr. Carl Nelson, we have continued the study of passively induced anaphylaxis, employing very large quantities of cortisone, 25 mgm daily for three days to 250 gm guinea pigs (28). With such high doses of cortisone there was a slight indication of a protective effect at the lowest antibody level (Table 3), which is hardly impressive. The failure of cortisone or ACTH to protect against anaphylaxis has been independently confirmed by Stoerk (29), Grabar, Benacerraf, and Biozzi (30), Malkiel (31), and Marcus and others (32).

Nelson, Fox, and Freeman (33) have reported that actively induced anaphylaxis in the mouse may be inhibited by 3 mgm cortisone daily, but not by 0.75 mgm. It is of interest that the protective effect of vaccination with dead tubercle bacilli in mice may be abolished by the administration of only 0.1 mgm cortisone daily, as was shown by Solotorovsky, Gregory, and Stoerk (34). This emphasizes some of the problems of relative pharmacological potency at different dosage quantities of the hormone, since thirty times as much was required for the inhibition of anaphylaxis. The inhibition by cortisone of a different type of anaphylactic death in adrenalectomized mice was reported by Dougherty (35). Larger shocking doses of horse serum were required by the actively immunized mice treated with cortisone than by those receiving no cortisone, the observation being interpreted as a degree of protection from anaphylaxis. As has been previously pointed out (1), however, protection from any noxious stimulus may be expected by substitution therapy in adrenalectomized animals. In addition, quantitative studies have repeatedly demonstrated that sensitivity reactions of the anaphylactic and Arthus types are far more sensitive to changes in the amount of antibody rather than of antigen, and for that reason passive immunization has been employed (1–2, 5, 28–32) to assure constant amounts of antibody and circumvent the inconstancy of anaphylaxis which may be caused by extreme variations of antibody level found in actively immunized animals.

TABLE 3
LACK OF EFFECT OF ADRENAL CORTICAL HORMONES ON ANAPHYLAXIS INDUCED IN GUINEA PIGS BY PASSIVE SENSITIZATION

SENSITIZING DOSE OF ANTIBODY NITROGEN—I.V.	LATENT PERIOD AND SHOCKING DOSE—I.V.	TREATED GROUP		UNTREATED GROUP
		Hormone Given before Shock	Severity of Shock	Severity of Shock
240 μg	1 hr. 0.16 mg Ea N.	2 mg ACTH 8 hrs. before	++++ ++ ++ ++	++++ ++++ +++ +++
30 μg	48 hrs. 0.16 mg Ea N.	2 mg ACTH q 6 h for 2 days	++++ ++++ ++++ +++ +++	++++ ++++ ++ +
32 μg	48 hrs. 0.06 mg Ea N. (gp. 300–400 Gm)	cortisone 2.5 mg I.M. for 3 days	+++ +++ +++ ++ ++	+++ +++ ++ ++ +
25 μg	48 hrs. 0.16 mg Ea N.	cortisone 25 mg I.M. for 4 days	++++ ++++ ++++ ++++ +++ +++	++++ ++++ ++++ ++++ ++++ ++
12.5 μg	48 hrs. 0.16 mg Ea N.	cortisone 25 mg I.M. for 4 days	++++ +++ ++ + + +	++++ ++++ ++++ ++++ ++++ +++

Experience with less-well-standardized allergic reactions, such as the tuberculin reaction, are more varied and apparently largely dependent on dosage and duration of hormone treatment. In animals and human beings made markedly hyperadrenal by ACTH or cortisone administration there appears to be a definite inhibition of the tuberculin reaction, which apparently results from altered skin reactivity rather than from any interference with an allergic reaction per se. A complete suppression of the guinea pig tuberculin reaction by ACTH was reported by Favour (36). Our experience has been that skin sensitivity to tuberculin or to streptococcal nucleoprotein was not altered in twenty patients receiving ACTH or cortisone in doses which were sufficient to cause a remission of their underlying disease process (1). However, in three instances of excessive hormone administration and marked hyperadrenalism with atrophic skin changes, inhibition of the tuberculin reaction did occur. In guinea pigs the tuberculin reaction was somewhat depressed, but by no means obliterated, by large doses of cortisone, that is, 25 mgm daily for several weeks (37).

It is difficult to ascribe the beneficial effect of cortisone or ACTH in clinical allergy simply to the inhibition of antibody production, except, perhaps, in a few instances of hemolytic anemias reported by Damashek (38). Generally the extent of inhibition of antibody, found in the rabbits studied by our group (3) and that of Germuth (5), is not appreciable enough to explain the dramatic clinical effects in which symptoms may disappear in a few hours. The failure of cortisone to inhibit experimentally induced allergic reaction is in marked contrast to the effects clinically observable in a variety of allergic diseases (39). The differences, however, may be due in part to the ameliorating effect of cortisone on inflamed tissue sites as opposed to its lack of effect when the inflammatory allergic reaction is induced in previously normal tissue. This may explain the discrepancy noted in patients with hayfever, in whom cortisone or ACTH may produce marked clinical remission of symptoms and signs of nasal congestion, but at the same time may fail to inhibit the reactivity of the patient's skin to an injection of ragweed extract. Such local variations in sensitivity may be attributed to the fact that different amounts of antibody are required for sensitization at different sites, but it is unlikely that cortisone lowers the antibody level rapidly enough to ameliorate symptoms at the site requiring a higher level of antibody for sensitization. The action of cortisone in such circumstances may then be on the various mesodermal cells of the inflamed site, fibroblasts, macrophages, eosinophiles, and others, and may have little to do with the inhibition of an allergic reaction per se. Tissue reactivity in granulating wounds and analogous lesions is observably depressed by cortisone (40), as is the edema in the Arthus reaction (41), despite the persistence of the final necrotizing effect (1, 5).

In summary, various aspects of the effect of ACTH and cortisone on the development of immune responses have been appraised. Antibody production is inhibited by those hormones during active immunization, after immunization is well established, and during the development of the secondary response. The failure of cortisone to affect the rate of disappearance of passively administered antibody and the timing of the effect of cortisone on the secondary response suggest that the synthesis of antibody is inhibited, as well as the "assimilation" of antigen.

Allergic reactions induced experimentally are not altered by cortisone or ACTH, despite the manifest amelioration observable in clinical allergic reactions. The interpretation of experimental and clinical studies are often complicated by variation in the dosage of the hormone, the types and amounts of antigen and antibody, and the animal species studied. Apparently cortisone does not inhibit the union of antigen and antibody nor the resulting sensitization reaction, but in large dosage may inhibit nonspecifically certain inflammatory reactions.

REFERENCES

1. Fischel, E. E., The relationship of adrenal cortical activity to immune responses, *Bull. N.Y. Acad. Med.*, 1950, 26:255.
2. Kabat, E. A., Quantitative immunochemical aspects of some allergic reactions, *Amer. J. Med.*, 1947, 3:535.
3. Bjørneboe, M., E. E. Fischel, and H. C. Stoerk, The effect of cortisone and adrenocorticotrophic hormone on the concentration of circulating antibody, *J. Exp. Med.*, 1951, 93:37.
4. Bjørneboe, M., and H. Gormsen, Experimental studies on the role of plasma cells as antibody producers, *Acta path. et microbiol. Scand.*, 1943, 20:649.
5. Germuth, F. G., Jr., and B. Ottinger, Effect of 17-hydroxy-11-dehydrocorticosterone (compound E) and of ACTH on Arthus reaction and antibody formation in the rabbit, *Proc. Soc. Exp. Biol. & Med.*, 1950, 74:815. Germuth, F. G., Jr., F. Oyama, and B. Ottinger, The mechanism of action of 17-hydroxy-11-dehydrocorticosterone (compound E) and of the adrenocorticotropic hormone on experimental hypersensitivity in rabbits, *J. Exp. Med.*, 1951, 94:139.
6. Havens, W. P., J. M. Shaffer, and C. J. Hopke, Jr., The effect of ACTH and cortisone on the concentration of circulating diphtheria antitoxin, *J. Immunol.*, 1952, 68:389.
7. Mirick, G. W., The effects of ACTH and cortisone on antibodies in human beings, *Bull. Johns Hopkins Hosp.*, 1951, 88:332.
8. Larson, D. L., and L. J. Tomlinson, Quantitative antibody studies in man; I: The effect of adrenal insufficiency and of cortisone on the level of circulating antibodies, *J. Clin. Invest.*, 1951, 30:1451.
9. Larson, D. L., and L. J. Tomlinson, *ibid.*, III: Antibody response in

leukemia and other malignant lymphomata. *J. Clin. Invest.*, 1953, 32:317.
10. Heidelberger, M., M. M. DiLapi, M. Siegel and A. W. Walter. Persistence of antibodies in human subjects injected with pneumococcal polysaccharide, *J. Immunol.*, 1950, 65:535.
11. Fischel, E. E., H. C. Stoerk, and M. Bjørneboe, Failure of cortisone to affect rate of disappearance of antibody protein, *Proc. Soc. Exp. Biol. & Med.*, 1951, 77:111.
12. Heidelberger, M., and E. A. Kabat, Chemical studies on bacterial agglutination; I: a method, *J. Exp. Med.*, 1934, 60:643.
13. Marshall, L. M., and F. Friedberg, Effect of ACTH on the incorporation of C^{14} of glycine in tissue proteins, *Endocrinol.*, 1951, 48:113.
14. Engel, F. L., General considerations concerning the role of the adrenal cortex in intermediary metabolism. This symposium, chapter 2.
15. Eisen, H. N., M. M. Mayer, D. H. Moore, R. Tarr, and H. C. Stoerk. Failure of adrenal cortical activity to influence circulating antibodies and gamma globulin, *Proc. Soc. Exp. Biol. & Med.*, 1947, 65:301.
16. Fischel, E. E., M. LeMay, and E. A. Kabat, The effect of adrenocorticotrophic hormone and X-ray on the amount of circulating antibody, *J. Immunol.*, 1949, 61:89.
17. De Vries, J. A., The effect of adrenocorticotrophic hormone on circulating antibody levels, *J. Immunol.*, 1950, 65:1.
18. Dougherty, T. F., J. H. Chase, and A. White, Pituitary-adrenal cortical control of antibody release from lymphocytes; an explanation of the anamnestic response, *Proc. Soc. Exp. Biol. & Med.*, 1945, 58:135.
19. Fischel, E. E., J. H. Vaughan, and C. Photopoulos, Inhibition of Rapid Production of Antibody by Cortisone. Study of Secondary Response, *Proc. Soc. Exp. Biol. & Med.*, 1952, 81:344.
20. Stoerk, H. C., Desoxypyridoxine observations in "acute pyridoxine deficiency," *Ann. N.Y. Acad. Sciences*, 1950, 52:1302.
21. Fagraeus, A., and K. Berglund, Personal communication and abstract, Section of Endocrinology, annual medical meetings, Stockholm, November, 1951.
22. Moeschlin, S., R. Baguena, and J. Baguena. Influence of ACTH and cortisone on the antibody production and the plasma cell reaction, *Bull. de L'Acad. Suisse des Sciences Medicales*, 1952, 8:153.
23. Kabat, E. A., A. Wolf, and A. E. Bezer, Studies on acute disseminated encephalomyelitis produced experimentally in rhesus monkeys; VII: The effect of cortisone, *J. Immunol.*, 1952, 68:265.
24. Kabat, E. A., A. Wolf, and A. E. Bezer, Studies on acute disseminated encephalomyelitis produced experimentally in rhesus monkeys, III, *J. Exp. Med.*, 1948, 88:417.
25. Rich, A. R., M. Berthrong, and I. L. Bennett, Jr., The effect of cortisone upon the experimental cardiovascular and renal lesions produced by anaphylactic hypersensitivity, *Bull. Johns Hopkins Hosp.*, 1950, 87: 549.

26. Cohen, S. G., and C. Moses, Effect of cortisone on experimental production of arteritis by passive sensitization, *J. Lab. Clin. Med.*, 1951, 37:764.
27. Leger, J., W. Leith, and B. Rose, effect of adrenocorticotrophic hormone. on anaphylaxis in the guinea pig, *Proc. Soc. Exp. Biol. & Med.*, 1948, 69:465.
28. Nelson, C. T., and E. E. Fischel. Unpublished data.
29. Stoerk, H. C. Inhibition of the tuberculin reaction by cortisone in vaccinated guinea pigs, *Fed. Proc.*, 1950, 9:345.
30. Grabar, P., B. Benacerraf, and G. Biozzi, Action de la cortisone et d'un extrait cortico-surrenal sur le choc anaphylactique passif du cobaye, *Annales de l'Inst. Pasteur*, 1951, 81:187.
31. Malkiel, S., The influence of ACTH and cortisone on histamine and anaphylactic shock in the guinea pig, *J. Immunol.*, 1951, 66:379.
32. Marcus, S., J. H. Carlquist, D. M. Donaldson and G. M. Christenson, Action of ACTH and cortisone on anaphylactic shock in the guinea pig, *Fed. Proc.*, 1952, 11:475.
33. Nelson, C. T., C. L. Fox, Jr., and E. B. Freeman, Inhibitory effect of cortisone on anaphylaxis in the mouse, *Proc. Soc. Exp. Biol. & Med.*, 1950, 75:181.
34. Solotorovsky, M., F. J. Gregory, and H. C. Stoerk, Loss of protection by vaccination following cortisone treatment in mice with experimentally induced tuberculosis, *Proc. Soc. Exp. Biol. & Med.*, 1951, 76:286.
35. Dougherty, T. F., The protective role of adrenal cortical secretion in the hypersensitive state. The Amer. Assoc. Advan. Science, Washington, D.C., 1950. Pituitary-Adrenal Function, p. 79.
36. Favour, C. B., cited by P. Forsham, in Proceedings of the First Clinical ACTH Conference. The Blakiston Company, Philadelphia, 1950, p. 520.
37. Fischel, E. E., E. A. Kabat, H. C. Stoerk, M. Skolnick and A. E. Bezer. Suppression by cortisone of granuloma formation and antibody in guinea pigs receiving egg albumin with Freund adjuvants, *Fed. Proc.*, 1953, 12: No. 1453.
38. Damashek, W., M. C. Rosenthal, and L. I. Schwartz, The treatment of acquired hemolytic anemia with adrenocorticotrophic hormone, *New England J. Med.*, 1951, 244:117.
39. Harvey, A. M., L. Shulman, and E. Shoenrich, The effect of ACTH and cortisone upon allergic diseases. This symposium, chapter 11.
40. Ragan, C., The effect of cortisone upon repair processes in dense and loose connective tissue. This symposium, chapter 5.
41. Humphrey, J. H., The effect of cortisone upon some experimental hypersensitivity reactions, *Brit. J. Exper. Path.*, 1951, 32:274.
42. Fischel, E. E., Hypersensitivity and the Hyperadrenal State, in C. Ragan, ed., Connective Tissues. Transactions of the Third Conference, Feb. 14–15, 1952. Josiah Macy, Jr., Foundation, N.Y.
43. Philips F. S., F. H. Hopkins, and M. L. H. Freeman, Effect of tris-(beta-chloroethyl) amine on antibody-production in goats, *J. Immunol.*, 1947, 55:289.

Chapter 7

DEPRESSION BY CORTISONE OF INHERITED AND ACQUIRED RESISTANCE TO INFECTION AND TO TUMOR GRAFTING

By HERBERT C. STOERK, *The Merck Institute for Therapeutic Research, Rahway, New Jersey*

MORE THAN TWENTY-FIVE YEARS AGO Murphy observed reduction of natural and of acquired resistance to experimental tuberculosis and to tumor grafting following X-radiation (1). This effect was ascribed by the author to the destructive action of the X-rays upon lymphocytes. This thesis has found ample support from several more recent studies in which loss of lymphoid tissue was produced by means other than X-radiation, including the induction, with cortisone or adrenocorticotrophic hormone, of the "hyperadrenal state."

Past experience has made it sufficiently evident that the integrity of lymphoid tissue is essential for the development of immune responses. Several agents causing striking loss of lymphoid cells were observed to inhibit antibody formation. X-ray (2), pyridoxine deprivation (3), nitrogen mustard (4), and antifolics (5) were shown to exert such an effect. Wells and Kendall (6) observed that injections of cortisone were followed by a striking reduction of lymphoid tissue. Subsequently it was found that the hyperadrenal state, with its attendant loss of lymphoid cells, is also associated with a depression of circulating antibody globulin (7–9) and with loss of resistance to a variety of infections (10–12).

The observations on cortisone-injected rats summarized below concern in part the loss of resistance to an unusual infection (Tyzzer's disease) attributed to *B. piliformis* (13). The susceptibility to this epizootic hepatitis was previously shown to be dependent upon genetic factors (14). In a somewhat similar fashion susceptibility to homologous tumor grafts is related to inherited properties. Suppression of "natural" and of acquired resistance to grafting with homologous tumor cells was also observed to follow treatment with cortisone.

The alterations by cortisone of the various tissue reactions which are thought to be related to the mechanism of defense against infection have been studied in some detail by several investigators. It appears difficult to draw general conclusions from these studies, because the results in each case depend upon the nature of the injuries inflicted, the species employed, and the dosage of cortisone used.

While it now seems unlikely that cortisone does affect the catabolism of protein in other tissues (15–16), apparently the breakdown of lymphoid cells is enhanced during the hyperadrenal state. Numerical estimation of mitotic activity in lymphoid tissue rendered atrophic through the action of cortisone, revealed undiminished mitotic activity (7). Furthermore, the uptake of labeled P was essentially unaltered in lymphoid cells of cortisone-treated animals (17). These findings indicate that cortisone causes degradation of lymphoid cells at an increased rate. Very large doses of cortisone in a short time caused nearly complete loss of the majority of mononuclear leucocytes in lymphoid organs and left almost exclusively a quantity of reticulo-endothelial or of epithelial syncytial cells. Sections of such greatly atrophied spleens of rodents contain megakaryoblasts and megakaryocytes, which together with the myeloid elements elsewhere remain unaffected. (18). Although cortisone fails to affect the granulocytes at the site of their formation, polymorphonuclear exudation is suppressed by large amounts of the steroid (19). Whether this results from the action of cortisone upon these cells under special circumstances or whether cortisone inhibits cellular exudation together with fluid exudation remains an open question. Furthermore, it was shown that in granulation tissue fibroblastic proliferation is inhibited during the hyperadrenal state (20–21). This action of cortisone is also likely to be a factor responsible for impairment of the defense mechanism. The doses necessary to obtain this inhibition are high, and it appears likely that this effect of cortisone is a consequence of its anti-anabolic action and is directed against the proliferation of the fibroblasts. The reticulo-endothelial system also is generally assumed to exert a protective action in infectious diseases. No valid tests have as yet been devised to measure its normal function, but the phagocytic activity of histiocytes may be judged to some extent. With respect to an apparently inert water-soluble material, carboxycellulose, the phagocytic activity of rats injected with cortisone was found to be strikingly increased (Fig. 1 A). However, enhancement of phagocytosis was less apparent when particulate matter (India ink) was injected with the cortisone.

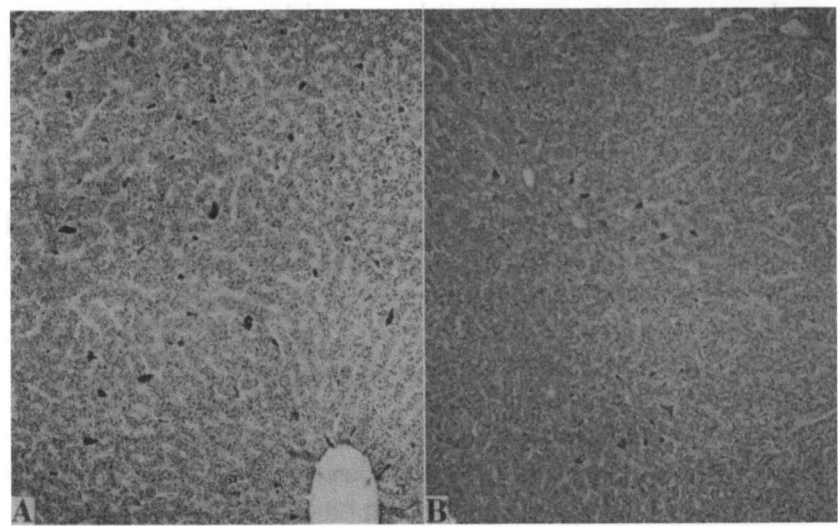

FIGURE 1. KUPFFER CELLS OF RATS INJECTED WITH SUSPENDING AGENT CONTAINING NA CARBOXY METHYL CELLULOSE
A. received 3 mg of cortisone daily for six weeks. B. received 3 mg of cholesterol daily for six weeks.

Therefore, the mononuclear leucocytes of the nonmyeloid series are apparently subject to increased destruction by cortisone, while the cells of the granulocytic and erythroid series, with mature histiocytes and mature fibroblasts, remain unaffected by its action. Although no data from comparative studies on this specific point are as yet available, our evidence indicates that the small lymphocytes are more readily suppressed by cortisone than are other mononuclear leucocytes.

When very large doses of cortisone (20–100 mg) were given daily to young rats (Table 1), the animals died after one to two weeks. Pre-

TABLE 1
EPIZOOTIC HEPATITIS IN CORTISONE-TREATED RATS

Number of Rats	Mg of Cortisone Injected Daily	Gm Body Initial	Weight Final	Days Survival Time Ave. (Range)	Incidence of Epizootic Hepatitis
3	20	117	76	14.5 (14–15)	3/3
3	50	102	70	9.5 (8–11)	2/3
3	100	115	77	7.5 (7–8)	1/3
10	30	117	74	12.3 (9–16)	9/10
10	30 [a]	117	83	21.2 (18–27)	1/10

[a] 2,000 units penicillin; 3,000 units streptomycin.

dominantly they succumbed to epizootic hepatitis (Tyzzer's disease) (Fig. 2 A and B), although many of them showed evidence of other infections as well. We have previously observed loss of resistance to epizootic hepatitis following nearly complete loss of lymphoid cells in "acute" pyridoxine deficiency (22). Earlier it was shown by Tyzzer and by Gowen and Schott that resistance to *B. piliformis* infection may be accounted for by a major genetic factor (14). In several of the animals there was also found a necrotizing gastritis (Fig. 2 C and D) reminiscent of the necrotizing esophagitis which is occasionally found in debilitated patients in association with *Candida albicans*. The rumen of such animals was heavily lined by a dense mixture of bacteria, although no *Candida albicans*-like organisms were encountered. Blood cultures of dying rats were taken, and in most cases they were found to contain a variety of microorganisms, among which hemolytic streptococci and *B. coli* were identified. In this connection it seems worthy of mention that morphological changes suggestive of viral invasion have been observed in other experiments. During a study concerning the Masugi nephritis of rats, intranuclear inclusions in renal tubular epithelia were found (Fig. 2 E) in rats injected with Upjohn's lipo adrenal extract (23) or with cortisone, but not in DCA-treated or uninjected animals.

From the above findings it became obvious that the mortality in rats treated with large doses of cortisone was at least partly caused by lowered resistance to infections and that the death from these intercurrent infectious diseases made it difficult to observe possible lethal toxic effects of the steroid itself. This was supported by the fact that antibiotics significantly prolonged the life of animals treated with massive doses of cortisone. The susceptibility of cortisone-injected animals to what appear to be saprophytes could have been caused by the elimination of any of the numerous undetermined factors which account for natural resistance. It appears more likely, however, that these findings concern selected instances in which acquired resistance, in a somewhat disguised form, is suppressed by the action of the steroid.

In view of findings showing that circulating antibodies are suppressed during the hyperadrenal state, it appeared likely that this effect, if sufficiently pronounced, should lead to loss of acquired resistance to infectious agents known to elicit measurable antibody formation.

An as yet undefined form of immunity distinct from the classic type, accounts for acquired resistance and hyperreactivity in tuberculosis. It was previously shown that the daily injection of 1 mg of cortisone over-

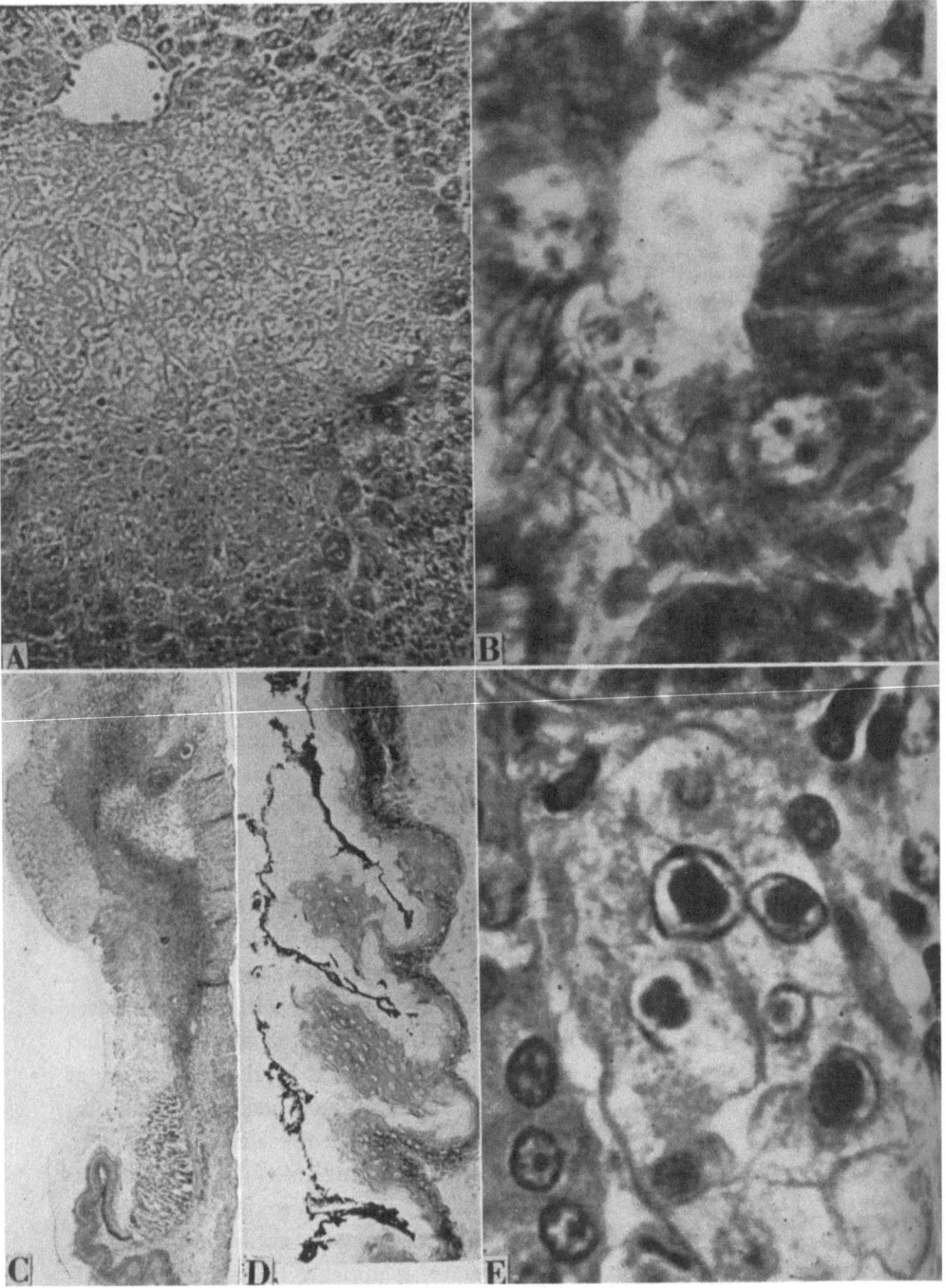

FIGURE 2.
A. Epizootic hepatitis (low power) area of necrosis in liver; B. *B. piliformis* (high power) in hepatic cells surrounding necrotic area; C. necrotizing gastritis in cortisone-injected rat; D. bacterial masses lining the rumen of rat stomach; E. intranuclear inclusions in epithelial cells of renal tubules.

came the beneficial effect of vaccination in mice infected with a highly virulent strain of *M. tuberculosis,* human type, but did not significantly enhance the lethality in nonvaccinated mice (24). It was also demonstrated that the tuberculin reactivity of sensitized guinea pigs is inhibited following a short treatment with cortisone. The data summarized in Fig. 3 illustrate this action of cortisone. The same treatment (at the

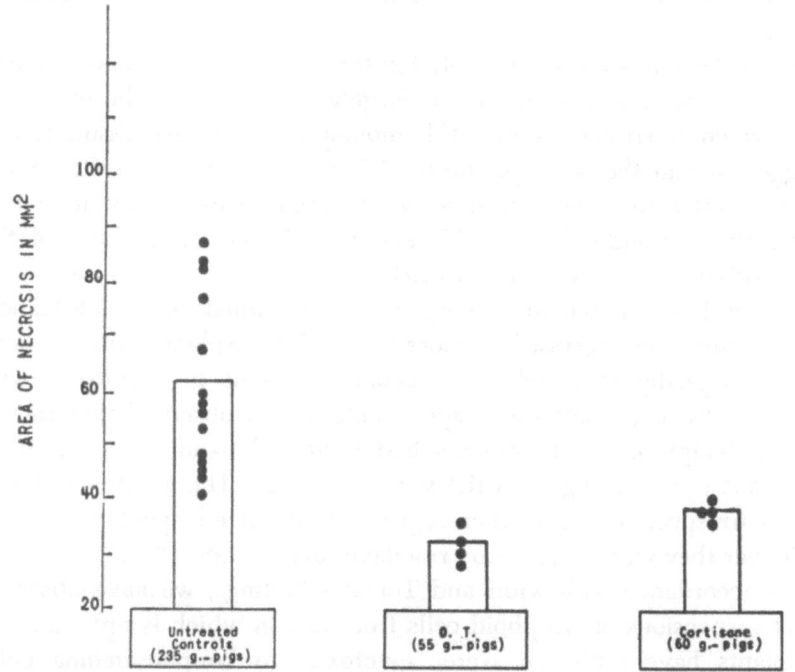

FIGURE 3. COMPARISON OF SIZE OF TUBERCULIN REACTIONS IN GROUPS OF 350 SENSITIZED GUINEA PIGS (EACH VALUE CORRESPONDING TO AN AVERAGE FROM 10-15 ANIMALS)

A single injection of old tuberculin 0.1 ccm or 5 daily injections of 5 mg of cortisone significantly depressed the size of the tuberculin reactions.

dose level employed) was found ineffective in suppressing established hypersensitivity of the "immediate" type (Arthus and anaphylaxis) (25) and therefore were apparently not caused by a nonspecific suppression of the reactivity of the skin or its supporting structures. It was shown by Landsteiner and Chase (26) that the "delayed" form of reactivity is transferable only by intact lymphoid cells, not by injured cells or serum. An immune principle sessile in intact lymphoid cells, strikingly resembling that of Landsteiner and Chase, was demonstrated by Kidd to be associated with acquired resistance to regrafting with neoplastic tissue (27). The finding that this type of immunity is also diminished when lymphoid tissue is suppressed by the administration of cortisone or by pyridoxine deprivation (28) points to another similarity between these two forms of immunity associated with "sensitized" cells.

It has been repeatedly suggested in the past that the success of grafting with homologous tumor tissue largely depends upon the same factors which determine the fate of homoio-grafts of normal tissue. It was suggested that the incompatibility of homologous tissue grafts among animals other than those of monozygotic origin is caused by undefined iso-antigens ("individuality differentials") distinct from those of the known blood group substances (29).

It has been known for a long time that animals in which tumor-transplants have regressed or those in which transplanted tumors have been surgically removed may become resistant to regrafting with tumor cells. From our own experiments it was observed that rats in which lymphosarcoma implants had regressed in all instances were resistant to regrafting with the same neoplasm. The resistance developed irrespective of whether regressions occurred spontaneously or whether they were induced by riboflavin deprivation (30).

In accordance with Kidd and Toolan's findings, we have observed that suspensions of lymphoid cells from rats in which lymphosarcoma implants have regressed were "cytotoxic" to lymphosarcoma cells. However, it was also seen that injections of normal, homologous lymphoid cells and to a lesser extent other tissues produced resistance to grafting with tumor cells (31). Repeated injections with homologous lymphoid cells "sensitized" the cells of the recipient rat against lymphosarcoma cells in apparently the same fashion as regressing tumor transplants (Fig. 4). Autologous lymphoid cells failed to produce resistance to tumor grafts, as did heterologous or injured homologous cells. No immune activity of serum could be demonstrated in rats immunized intensely with homologous lymphoid cells. These findings apparently indicate that intact lymphoid cells more than other cells carry certain iso-antigens ("individuality differentials") which in a population of animals genetically more different than monozygotic individuals gave rise to immune responses. The main sites of this immunity, at least as far as available for circulation, appear to be the lymphoid cells of the recipient animal.

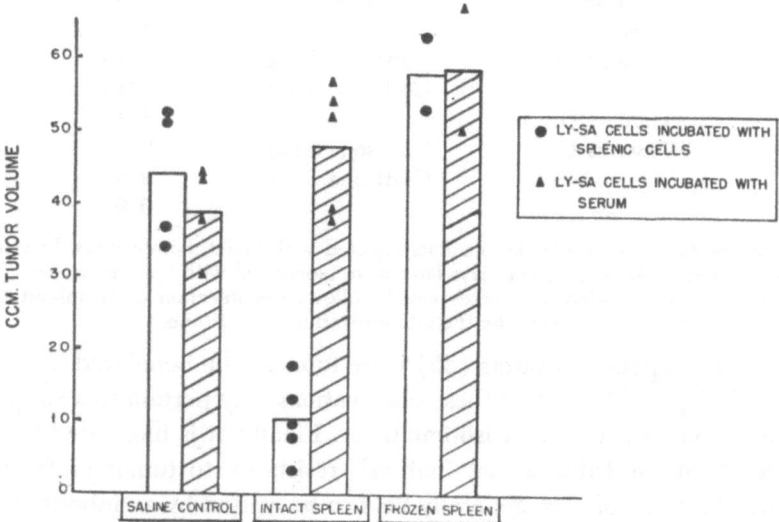

FIGURE 4. SENSITIZATION OF SPLENIC CELLS OF RATS INJECTED WITH INTACT HOMOLOGOUS SPLEEN

Three groups of 8-15 rats each were injected 3× weekly one with suspensions of intact, homologous, splenic cells, the other with an identical suspension subjected to freezing and thawing and the third with saline. One week after the last injection pools of serum and of saline suspended lymphoid cells (spleen) from those 3 groups of rats were tested for their "cytotoxic" action upon lymphosarcoma cells. 250,000 lymphosarcoma cells were mixed with the respective material, incubated at 37°C for one hour, and then injected into groups of 6 susceptible rats. Each point on the graph represents the average tumor volume attained 14 days after the inoculation.

From the experiments summarized in Table 2 it may be seen that the acquired resistance to grafting with lymphosarcoma cells is diminished when, following the injection of homologous lymphoid cells, cortisone is administered prior to the challenging inoculation. Recently it was observed that the administration of cortisone prolongs the persistence of homologous transplants of skin (32) and of kidney (33), as it was also reported to counteract the ill effects of incompatible transfusions. Furthermore, diseases such as certain hemolytic anemias (34) and

TABLE 2

SUPPRESSION OF RESISTANCE TO GRAFTING BY CORTISONE

Cell Suspension Injected [a]	Treatment after Injection	Number of Takes
Spleen (i.v.)	...	3/9
Spleen (i.v.)	Cortisone 5 mg	7/10
...	Cortisone 5 mg	10/10
Thymus (i.v.)	...	3/10
Thymus (i.v.)	Cortisone 5 mg	9/9
...	Cortisone 5 mg	9/9
...	...	9/9

[a] Seven days before inoculation. Rats injected with intact, homologous, lymphoid cells (spleen or thymus) seven days later were inoculated with lymphosarcoma. The greatly lowered incidence of takes which follows the injection of lymphoid cells was nearly restored to normal by the administration of cortisone.

thrombocytopenic purpuras (35) were found to be benefitted by cortisone. It is possible that all these observations may pertain to a suppression of some such form of iso-immunity. Finally, it is illustrated by the experiments in Table 3 that "natural" resistance to tumor grafting in some of a stock of rats, generally held to be caused by an inherited iso-immunological incompatibility, may be suppressed by the administration of cortisone.

An agent capable of suppressing immune responses without causing irreversible systemic damage has in the past been suggested to be of

TABLE 3

SUPPRESSION OF "NATURAL" RESISTANCE TO TUMOR GRAFTING BY CORTISONE

Group	Mg Cortisone	Number of Rats [a]	Number of Regressions
I	2	38	1
II	3	18	0
III	5	26	0
I–III	2–5	82	1 (1.2%)
IV	—	38	8
V	—	18	7
VI	—	26	10
IV–VI	—	82	25 (30.5%)

[a] Of 164 rats inoculated with lymphosarcoma, half were injected daily with cortisone. Twenty-five spontaneous regressions occurred in the untreated group, while only one rat in the cortisone-treated group failed to die with a large tumor.

potential therapeutic value in combatting diseases of hypersensitivity (36). Since it was discovered by Hench and Kendall that rheumatoid arthritis and other conditions strongly suspected to be of allergic etiology were alleviated by cortisone, it has been considered by some that this may be caused by a suppression of immunity by cortisone. It has become evident that cortisone or adrenocorticotrophin suppress the formation of antibodies of the classic type without altering their rate of disappearance. Immune principles, such as that of Landsteiner and Chase and that of Kidd, are dependent for their persistence upon the integrity of the lymphoid cells. Since the latter are actively destroyed during the hyperadrenal state, it appears logical that adrenal cortical hyperactivity should not only interfere with the formation of such immune principles but also aid in their actual destruction. This could represent a relevant factor in the suppression by cortisone of certain types of hypersensitivity.

REFERENCES

1. Murphy, J. B., The Lymphocytic in Resistance to Tissue Grafting, Malignant Disease and Tuberculous Infection. Monographs of the Rockefeller Institute for Medical Research, 1926.
2. Wilson, G. W., and A. A. Miles, Principles of Bacteriology and Immunology, Topley and Wilson, The Williams & Wilkins Co., Baltimore, 1946.
3. Stoerk, H. C., and H. N. Eisen, Suppression of circulation antibodies in pyridoxine deficiency, *Proc. Soc. Exp. Biol. & Med.*, 1946, 62:88.
4. Philips, F. S., F. H. Hopkins, and M. L. H. Freeman, Effect of tris-(beta-chloroethyl) amine on antibody-production in goats, *J. Immunol.*, 1947, 55:289.
5. Oleson, J. J., Studies on pteroylglutamic acid inhibitors, *Trans. of N.Y. Acad. of Sci.*, 1950, 12:118.
6. Wells, B. B., and E. G. Kendall, The Influence of Corticosterone and 17-Hydroxy-11-Dehydrocorticosterone on Somatic Growth, *Proc. Staff Meet. Mayo Clinic*, 1940, 15:324.
7. Stoerk, H. C., and M. Solotorovsky, Adrenal cortical activity in relation to lymphoid tissue and to immune bodies, *Am. J. Path.*, 1950, 26:708.
8. Germuth, F. G., and B. Ottinger, Effect of 17-Hydroxy-11-Dehydrocorticosterone (Compound E) and of ACTH on Arthus Reaction and Antibody Formation in the Rabbit, *Proc. Soc. Exp. Biol. & Med.*, 1950, 74:815.
9. Bjørneboe, M., E. E. Fischel, and H. C. Stoerk, The Effect of Cortisone and Adrenocorticotrophic Hormone on the Concentration of Circulating Antibody, *J. Exp. Med.*, 1951, 93:37.
10. Kass, E. H., S. H. Ingbar, and M. Finland, Effects of adrenocorticotropic

hormone in pneumonia; clinical, bacteriological and serological studies, *Ann. Int. Med.*, 1950, 33:1081.
11. Schwartzman, G., Enhancing effect of cortisone upon poliomyelitis infection (strain MEF1) in hamsters and mice, *Proc. Soc. Exp. Biol. & Med.*, 1950, 75:835.
12. Robinson, H. J., Effects of cortisone on intradermal pneumococcal infections in rabbits, *Fed. Proc.*, 1951, 10:332.
13. Tyzzer, E. E., A fatal disease of the Japanese waltzing mouse caused by a sporebearing bacillus (*Bacillus piliformis*), *J. Med. Res.*, 1917, 37:307.
14. Gowen, J. W., and R. G. Schott, (a) Genetic predisposition to *Bacillus piliformis* infection among mice, *J. Hyg.* (Camb.) 1933 (a), 33:370.
15. Clark, I., Effect of cortisone on protein metabolism in the rat as studied with isotopic glycine, *Fed. Proc.*, 1951, 9:161.
16. Fischel, E. E., H. C. Stoerk, and M. Bjørneboe. Failure of cortisone to affect rate of disppearance of antibody protein, *Proc. Soc. Exp. Biol. & Med.*, 1951, 77:111.
17. Clark, I., and H. C. Stoerk. Not yet published.
18. Gordon, A. S., S. J. Piliero, and D. Landaw, Influence of adrenal factors in hemopoiesis in the rat, *J. Clin. Endocrinol.*, 1951, 11:772 (Inc. Soc. Proc.).
19. Taubenhaus, M., and G. D. Amromin, The effects of the hypophysis, thyroid, sex steroids and the adrenal cortex upon granulation tissue, *J. Lab. & Clin. Med.*, 1950, 36:7.
20. Plotz, C. M., E. L. Howes, J. W. Blunt, K. Meyer, and C. Ragan. Action of cortisone on mesenchymal tissues, *Arch. Dermat. & Syph.*, 1950, 61:919.
21. Baker, B. L., and W. L. Whitaker, Interference with wound healing by the bacterial action of adrenalcortical steroids, *Endocrinology*, 1950, 46:544.
22. Stoerk, H. C., Desoxypyridoxine; observations in "acute pyridoxine deficiency," *Ann. N.Y. Acad. Sci.*, 1949, 52:1302.
23. Knowlton, A. I., H. C. Stoerk, B. C. Seegal, and E. N. Loeb. Influence of adrenal cortical steroids upon the blood pressure and the rate of progression of experimental nephritis in rats, *Endocrinology*, 1946, 38:315.
24. Solotorovsky, M., F. J. Gregory, and H. C. Stoerk, Loss of protection by vaccination following cortisone treatment in mice with experimentally induced tuberculosis, *Proc. Soc. Exp. Biol. & Med.*, 1951, 76:286.
25. Stoerk, H. C., Inhibition of the tuberculin reaction by cortisone in vaccinated guinea pigs, *Fed. Proc.*, 1950, 9:345.
26. Landsteiner, K., and M. W. Chase, Experiments on transfer of cutaneous sensitivity to simple compounds, *Proc. Soc. Exp. Biol. & Med.*, 1942, 49:688.
27. Kidd, J. G., and H. W. Toolan, Effects of "sensitized" lymphocytes on transplanted cancer cells, *Fed. Proc.*, 1950, 9:385.

28. Stoerk, H. C., Suppression of tumor immunity by cortisone and following pyridoxine deprivation, *Proc. Am. Cancer Society* (ACTH-Cortisone Conference, October, 1950, New York).
29. Loeb, L. The Biological Basis of Individuality. Charles C. Thomas, Springfield, Ill., 1945.
30. Stoerk, H. C., and G. A. Emerson, Complete regression of lymphosarcoma implants following temporary induction of riboflavin deficiency in mice, *Proc. Soc. Exp. Biol. & Med.*, 1949, 70:703.
31. Stoerk, H. C., T. Budzilovich, and T. C. Bielinski, Resistance to grafting with lymphosarcoma cells in rats injected with homologous lymphoid cells, *J. Mount Sinai Hospital*, 1952, 19:169.
32. Billingham, R. E., P. L. Krohn, and P. B. Medawar, Effect of cortisone on survival of skin homograft in rabbits, *Brit. Med. J.*, 1951, 1:1157.
33. Simonsen, M. Personal communication.
34. Dameshek, W., M. C. Rosenthal, and L. I. Schwartz, The Treatment of acquired hemolytic anemia with adrenocorticotrophic hormone, *New England J. Med.*, 1951, 244:117.
35. Faloon, W. W., R. W. Greene, and E. L. Lozner, The hemostatic effect in thrombocytopenia as studied by the use of ACTH and cortisone, *J. Clin. Invest.*, 1951, 30:638.
36. Stoerk, H. C. Effects of calcium deficiency and pyridoxine deficiency on thymic atrophy (accidental involution), *Proc. Soc. Exp. Biol. & Med.*, 1946, 62:90.

Chapter 8

CONSTITUTIONAL FACTORS IN RESISTANCE TO INFECTION; THE EFFECT OF CORTISONE ON THE PATHOGENESIS OF TUBERCULOSIS [1]

By Max B. Lurie, Peter Zappasodi, Arthur M. Dannenberg, Jr.,[2] and Eugenia Cardona-Lynch, *The Henry Phipps Institute, University of Pennsylvania, Philadelphia, Pa.*

In the study of the role of sex hormones in resistance to infection (1–2), it was noted that tuberculosis in rabbits is accompanied by a marked hypertrophy of the adrenal cortex. Furthermore, it has been observed that the weight of the adrenals of the genetically most resistant race is greater than that of a susceptible race following a tuberculous infection, Table 1. Therefore, investigations on the role of the adrenal cortex in resisting the disease were undertaken, to determine whether by increasing adrenal function resistance can be increased and, conversely, whether by lowering this function the native resistance can be diminished.

When genetically susceptible and resistant rabbits inhale a certain number of virulent human-type tubercle bacilli, an extensive pulmonary tuberculosis results, as a rule, five months after infection in the former and not at all in the latter (3). If rabbits thus quantitatively exposed are killed five weeks after infection, the number of primary tubercles found in these two types of animals is inversely proportional to their genetic resistance; the greater the resistance, the fewer the primary pulmonary foci (4).

METHODS AND MATERIALS

When synthetic cortisone became available, the following experiment was performed. Twenty litter mates of the genetically uniform and highly susceptible strain, FC, were divided into two groups of ten each. They were placed in a room at a constant temperature of

---

[1] Aided by grants from the Commonwealth Fund, the National Tuberculosis Association and the Federal Security Agency, Public Health Service.

[2] Charles Hartwell Cocke Memorial Fellow of the National Tuberculosis Association.

TABLE 1

WEIGHT OF ADRENALS IN SUSCEPTIBLE RACE FC AND RESISTANT RACE III RABBITS 32–37 DAYS AFTER THE SIMULTANEOUS INHALATION OF VIRULENT HUMAN TYPE TUBERCLE BACILLI, H37Rv

DURATION OF INFECTION IN DAYS	RABBIT NUMBER		NUMBER OF TUBERCLES IN LUNGS OF		WEIGHT OF ADRENALS IN MG/100 gm OF BODY WEIGHT	
	FC	III	FC	III	FC	III
32	FC 2–9	III 3–26	107	4	11	15
35	FC 3=14	III 3=2	14	0	10	14
35	FC 3=4	III 1–V37	25	0	14	34
35	FC 3=13	III 3–10	60	2	8	20
35	FC 3=19	III 2–1	19	2	20	19
35	FC 2–29	III 2–6	2	2	6	15
35–37	FC 3=12	III 2–2	115	13	11	22
35–37	FC 3=33	III 2–7	79	1	10	34
35–37	FC 2–53	...	40	...	8	...
35–37	FC 3=16	III 3–3	87	32	15	18
35–37	FC 3=28	III 3–24	131	7	12	19
35–37	FC 3=40	III 3–40	69	5	11	18
Mean			62 ± 12	6 ± 3	11 ± 1	21 ± 2
				CR = 4.4		CR = 4.5
				P = 0.000		P = 0.000

$21 \pm 2°$ C. Total and differential counts of their blood cells and their fasting blood sugar were determined. At the same time the spread of India ink and of rabbit hemoglobin in the skin was measured four hours after injection. The inflammation at the site of injection of these substances in the skin was ascertained on the following day. Having obtained these base lines, ten of the rabbits were given 2 mg of cortisone acetate per kilo, intramuscularly, on alternate days. The ten control litter mates received the same amount of the suspending medium without the cortisone and by the same route at the same time intervals. Three days after the beginning of cortisone treatment, when the absolute number of circulating lymphocytes in the blood of the experimental animals had been markedly depressed and when the fasting blood sugar of the same animals had increased by comparison with the essentially unchanged levels of these items in the control animals, both groups were simultaneously exposed to inhalation of known numbers of viable, virulent, human-type tubercle bacilli, H37Rv, in the apparatus for experimental airborne infection previously described (5).

After the control and experimental animals were infected, the cortisone and the suspending medium, respectively, were administered to each group at the same intervals and in the same amounts, as stated above, throughout the course of the experiment. During this time the absolute number of circulating lymphocytes of the blood, the fasting blood sugar, the blood ascorbic acid, the development of tuberculin sensitivity and antibodies against the tubercle bacillus, the spread of India ink and rabbit hemoglobin in the skin, and the inflammation induced by these agents in this tissue were measured.

As may be seen in Table 2, the absolute number of circulating lymphocytes of the cortisone-treated animals diminished continuously in statistically significant amounts in the course of treatment, while that of the controls actually increased as compared with the base lines. Likewise, the fasting blood sugar of the experimental animals increased under treatment, while in the controls this increment was much smaller.

Table 3 shows that the spread of India ink, or hemoglobin, in the skin was not definitely affected in either the control or the experimental animals. However, the inflammation induced by these agents in the skin

TABLE 2

THE EFFECT OF CORTISONE ON THE CIRCULATING LYMPHOCYTES, ON TWO INTERVALS FOLLOWING TREATMENT

RABBIT NUMBER		ORIGINAL ABSOLUTE NUMBER OF LYMPHOCYTES, MM^3		PERCENTAGE OF ORIGINAL NUMBER OF LYMPHOCYTES IN BLOOD AFTER 3 DAYS OF TREATMENT		PERCENTAGE OF ORIGINAL NUMBER OF LYMPHOCYTES IN BLOOD AFTER 25 DAYS OF TREATMENT AND 21 DAYS AFTER INFECTION	
Non-treated	Treated	Non-treated	Treated	Non-treated	Treated	Non-treated	Treated
C 11	E 1	4,200	2,940	107	35	77	16
C 12	E 2	2,490	4,470	202	36	175	23
C 13	E 3	2,180	3,920	103	44	147	33
C 14	E 4	5,060	2,950	75	65	102	69
C 15	E 5	4,930	3,360	86	49	99	35
C 16	E 6	4,340	4,320	89	61	96	16
C 17	E 7	4,020	4,030	133	82	85	32
C 18	E 8	3,480	6,360	145	53	173	20
C 19	E 9	3,420	5,180	113	58	132	40
C 20	E 10	10,060	4,810	66	52	67	25
Mean		4,418	4,234	112 ± 12	54 ± 4	115 ± 12	31 ± 5
					CR = 4.6		CR = 6.7
					P = 0.000		P = 0.000

TABLE 3

THE EFFECT OF CORTISONE ON THE SPREAD OF INDIA INK AND RABBIT HEMO-
GLOBIN IN THE SKIN AND ON THE INFLAMMATORY RESPONSE OF THE
CONNECTIVE TISSUE TO THESE SUBSTANCES

NUMBER OF RABBITS		SPREAD				INFLAMMATION			
		India Ink, 4 Hrs.		Hemoglobin, 4 Hrs.		India Ink, 1 Day		Hemoglobin, 1 Day	
Non-treated	Treated	Non-treated mm^2	Treated mm^2	Non-treated mm^2	Treated mm^2	Non-treated mm^3	Treated mm^3	Non-treated mm^3	Treated mm^3
10	10	714	724	667	725	586 ± 50	291 ± 22	266 ± 38	115 ± 16
							$P = 0.000$		$P = 0.001$

TABLE 4

THE EFFECT OF CORTISONE ON THE DEVELOPMENT OF THE TUBERCULIN
REACTION IN THE SKIN AT DIFFERENT INTERVALS FOLLOWING THE
INHALATION OF HUMAN TYPE TUBERCLE BACILLI

RABBIT NUMBER		INFLAMMATION, MM^3 16–18 DAYS AFTER INFECTION		INFLAMMATION, MM^3 21 DAYS AFTER INFECTION		INFLAMMATION, MM^3 25–27 DAYS AFTER INFECTION	
Non-treated	Treated	Non-treated	Treated	Non-treated	Treated	Non-treated	Treated
C 11	E 1	13	0	288	0	391	14
C 12	E 2	17	0	126	12	175	23
C 13	E 3	7	0	530	26	608	14
C 14	E 4	10	0	216	16	288	27
C 15	E 5	95	0	152	0	315	21
C 16	E 6	6	0	54	0	240	10
C 17	E 7	0	0	18	0	68	14
C 18	E 8	8	0	190	0	373	11
C 19	E 9	11	0	92	11	152	21
C 20	E 10	0	0	15	0	83	0
Mean		17 ± 8	0	168 ± 47	7 ± 3	269 ± 49	16 ± 2
			$P = 0.025$		$P = 0.001$		$P = 0.000$

was markedly reduced in the experimental animals as compared with the control animals, the results being statistically significant. Likewise, as may be seen from Table 4, tuberculin produced much more inflammation in the control rabbits than in the cortisone-treated rabbits. This is clearly because of the protective effect exercised by cortisone on the capillaries against agents which increase their permeability, as was observed by Menkin (6). Peptone, which releases fibrinolysin in vitro, increases the permeability of the capillaries of normal rabbits to a much greater extent than it does in cortisone-treated animals. Moreover, pure fibrinolysin, a substance released at sites of inflammation (7), causes marked leakage from the vessels of normal rabbits and scarcely affects cortisone-treated animals when injected into the skin. Furthermore, the capillary fragility of cortisone-treated rabbits is much less than that of untreated controls, as was indicated by capillary hemorrhage induced by applying uniform suction to the skin. These observations indicate that cortisone not only protects the capillary wall against chemical agents which disrupt its integrity but also that the tensile strength of the wall against the internal blood pressure is augmented by the hormone.

The antibody production against the tubercle bacillus, as revealed by the Middlebrook and Dubos hemagglutination test (8), was not conspicuously affected, although the titer in the experimental animals was slightly, though uniformly, lower than in the controls.

It was previously demonstrated by Gordon and Katsh (9) that starvation increases the phagocytic activity of macrophages by stimulating the adrenal function. In view of this finding, the following experiment was deemed advisable. On the thirty-fourth and thirty-sixth days of infection one half of the experimental and the control rabbits were given an intravenous injection of 6 cc. per kilo of a 1:3 saline dilution of India ink, and were killed by air embolism three hours later. Another group of three cortisone-treated and three untreated rabbits were similarly injected and were killed two weeks after infection. Their livers and spleens were digested with concentrated KOH, and the weight of contained carbon was determined. Histological sections of these organs were also studied. It was found that the phagocytosis of carbon particles and tubercle bacilli was markedly increased in the cortisone-treated animals (Figs. 1–2). The remaining rabbits were killed thirty-five or thirty-eight days after inhalation of tubercle bacilli. Each cortisone-treated rabbit was killed on the same day following infection as was its control litter mate infected under identical conditions. All animals were starved for seventeen hours before they were killed. The glycogen present in the livers and the weights of the liver, spleen, adrenals, gonads, and pituitary of all control and experimental animals were determined.

It was found (Table 5) that the livers of the cortisone-treated rab-

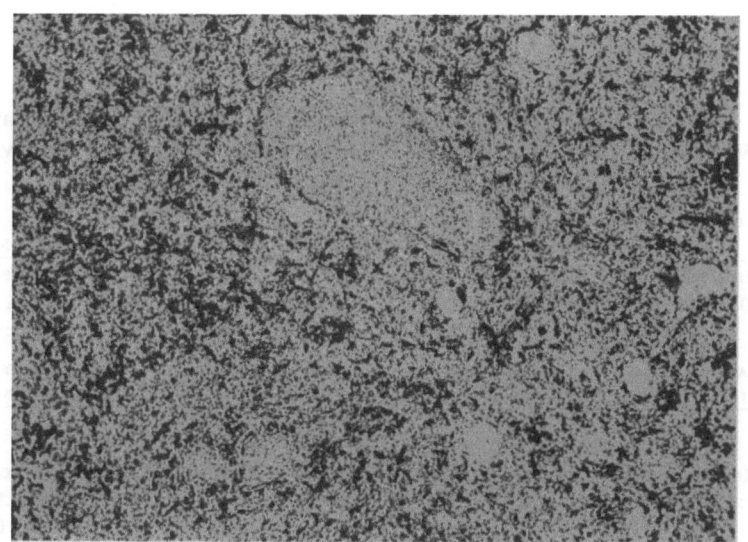

FIGURE 1. THE PHAGOCYTOSIS OF CARBON IN AN UNTREATED RABBIT TWO WEEKS AFTER INHALATION INFECTION, SHOWING INTACTNESS OF THE LYMPHOCYTES IN THE LYMPH FOLLICLES OF THE SPLEEN

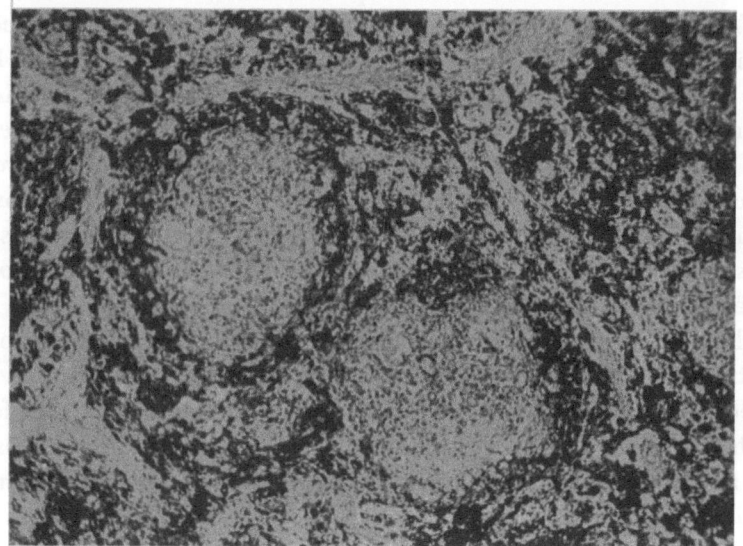

FIGURE 2. PHAGOCYTOSIS OF CARBON BY THE MACROPHAGES OF THE SPLEEN IN A CORTISONE-TREATED ANIMAL INFECTED AT THE SAME TIME AS THE RABBIT SHOWN IN FIG. 1, SHOWING INTENSE PHAGOCYTOSIS OF CARBON BY A BASKET-LIKE NETWORK OF THE MACROPHAGES AND RETICULAR CELLS AROUND THE FOLLICLES AND DISINTEGRATION OF LYMPHOCYTES

TABLE 5

The Weight of Organs of Cortisone-Treated and Control Litter Mates of the FC Family 34–38 Days Following Quantitative Inhalation of Human Type Tubercle Bacilli

NUMBER OF RABBITS		BODY WEIGHT GM		LIVER GM/100 GM		SPLEEN MG/100 GM	
Control	Treated	Control	Treated	Control	Treated	Control	Treated
10	10	3,024	2,858	2 ± 0.09	4.8 ± 0.29	53 ± 3	31 ± 2
					P = 0.000		P = 0.000

ADRENALS MG/100 GM		THYROID MG/100 GM		TESTES MG/100 GM		PITUITARY MG/100 GM	
				Six Control Rabbits	Seven Treated Rabbits		
Control	Treated	Control	Treated			Control	Treated
12.8 ± 1	6.6 ± 0.6	4.7 ± 0.13	4 ± 0.05	148 ± 6	71.4 ± 9.6	0.8 ± 0.06	0.7 ± 0.05
	P = 0.000		P = 0.000		P = 0.000		P = 0.120

bits were twice as heavy as those of the controls. This was because of excessive deposits of glycogen and fat in the markedly enlarged liver cells of the experimental animals, obviously resulting from the physiological effects of the cortisone. The spleens of the cortisone rabbits were markedly reduced in weight, as a result of the lympholytic effect of cortisone, demonstrable even two weeks after infection (Figs. 1–2). The adrenals were markedly atrophied in the experimental animals, clearly because of the high level of cortisone in their blood. There was also marked atrophy of the male gonads, though the ovaries were not affected. The thyroids of the experimental rabbits were uniformly, though only moderately, reduced in weight. It is clear from these results that the experimental animals were under the intense physiological effects of cortisone.

The number and size of the tubercles developed in the lungs of the control and experimental rabbits were accurately determined and are listed in Table 6. It will be noted that the number of tubercles found in the cortisone rabbits was uniformly greater than in the controls. On the average, three to four times as many tubercles resulted from the inhalation of human tubercle bacilli in cortisone-treated rabbits as from the inhalation of the same numbers of bacilli by untreated litter mates of the same inbred strain and the same genetic resistance to the infection (Fig. 3). This difference is statistically significant.

However, the size of the individual tubercles in the lung was uniformly and markedly smaller in the cortisone-treated animals. Further-

TABLE 6

The Effect of Cortisone on the Ratio between the Number of Human Type Tubercle Bacilli Inhaled and the Number of Pulmonary Tubercles Generated in FC Rabbits 34 to 38 Days after Infection

RABBIT NUMBER		NUMBER OF TUBERCLES		SIZE OF TUBERCLES MM		NUMBER OF VIABLE BACILLI YIELDING ONE TUBERCLE	
Control	Cortisone	Control	Cortisone	Control	Cortisone	Control	Cortisone
FC 2–46	FC 2=1	55	159	6	2	81	39
FC 2–47	FC 2–49	63	142	5	2	95	40
FC 3=18	FC 3=24	201	241	5	3	30	21
FC 2–50	FC 2–51	72	275	5	3	92	24
FC 3=29	FC 3=30	32	131	5	4	226	54
FC 3=31	FC 3=32	17	47	6	3	105	38
FC 4=3	FC 4=2	8	71	Large	Small	265	25
FC 3=37	FC 3=35	36	36	5	Small	44	38
FC 3=36	FC 3=39	9	43	6	2	160	34
FC 2–56	FC 2–55	11	40	7	1	98	36
Mean						120 ± 22	35 ± 2.9
						$P = 0.002$	

more, the spread of the disease to the draining tracheobronchial lymph nodes (Table 7) and to the internal organs was markedly smaller in the experimental rabbits.

It was also found in these experiments and in others not detailed here that initially, notwithstanding the demonstrated greater in vivo phagocytic capacity afforded the reticulo-endothelial cells by cortisone, the number of inhaled bacilli arrested in the lung of the experimental rabbits was no greater than that retained by the controls. Two weeks after infection the bacilli were more numerous in the lungs of the cortisone rabbits, as was observed both histologically and by culture (Figs.

TABLE 7

Number of Tubercle Bacilli Cultured from 2 mg of Lung and from Draining Tracheobronchial Nodes of Control and Cortisone-Treated Rabbits Two Weeks after Simultaneous Inhalation of Human Type Tubercle Bacilli

RABBIT NUMBER		LUNGS		TRACHEOBRONCHIAL NODES	
Control	Experimental	Control	Experimental	Control	Experimental
Ca 5=10	Ca 5=9	103	877	21	2.0
Ca 5=21	Ca 5=20	191	360	30	9
Ca 5=19	Ca 5–47	224	305	68	0.7

4–5). However, in the draining tracheobronchial lymph nodes of the controls they greatly outnumbered those of the experimental animals. Five weeks after exposure the pulmonary lesions in the cortisone rabbits were sharply demarcated foci of caseous pneumonia with intra-

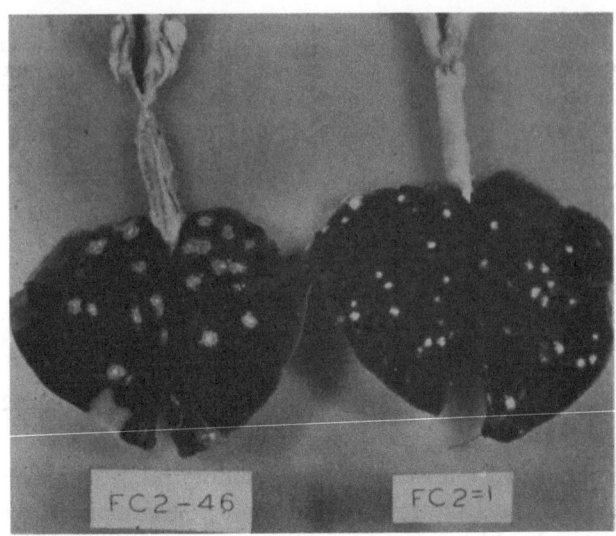

FIGURE 3. THE LUNGS OF CONTROL RABBIT FC 2-46 AND OF CORTISONE-TREATED RABBIT FC $2 = 1$, BOTH OF WHICH INHALED FOUR TO SIX THOUSAND HUMAN-TYPE TUBERCLE BACILLI, H37Rv

Both were killed thirty-four days following infection. In the control rabbit (FC 2-46) 81 inhaled bacilli generated a pulmonary focus, while in the experimental rabbit (FC $2 = 1$) 39 tubercle bacilli sufficed to generate a pulmonary tubercle. The average diameter of the tubercles was 6 and 2 mm, respectively. Note consolidation of the lung tissue around the caseous centers in the normal animal and absence of perifocal inflammation about the whiter caseous sites in the cortisone-treated animal. Both lungs were blackened by simultaneous intravenous injection of India ink.

alveolar plugs of partially caseated cells swarming with inordinate numbers of bacilli (Figs. 6–8). There was little interstitial or perifocal inflammation. These caseous plugs were largely out of contact with the circulation. The lesions in the controls were tuberculous granulomas, with well-advanced, discrete caseous centers and moderate numbers of bacilli surrounded by widely spreading zones of infiltrating perifocal

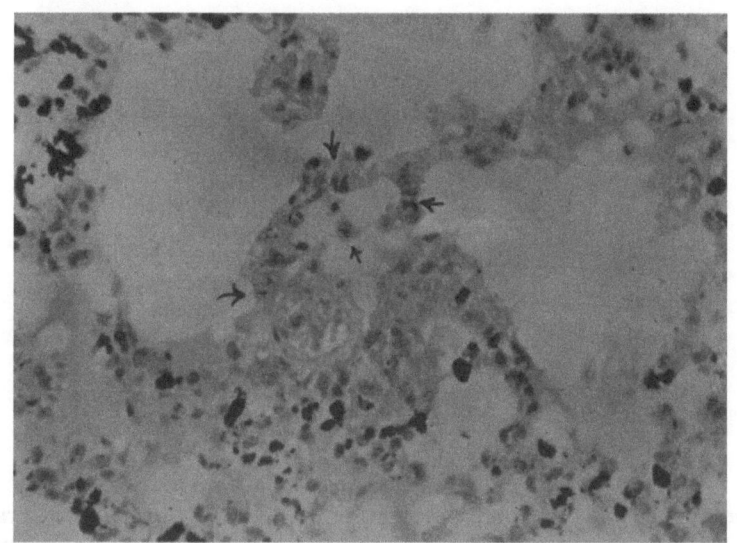

FIGURE 4. PRIMITIVE LESION IN AN UNTREATED RABBIT TWO WEEKS AFTER THE INHALATION OF TUBERCLE BACILLI, SHOWING TUBERCLE BACILLI INSIDE MACROPHAGES

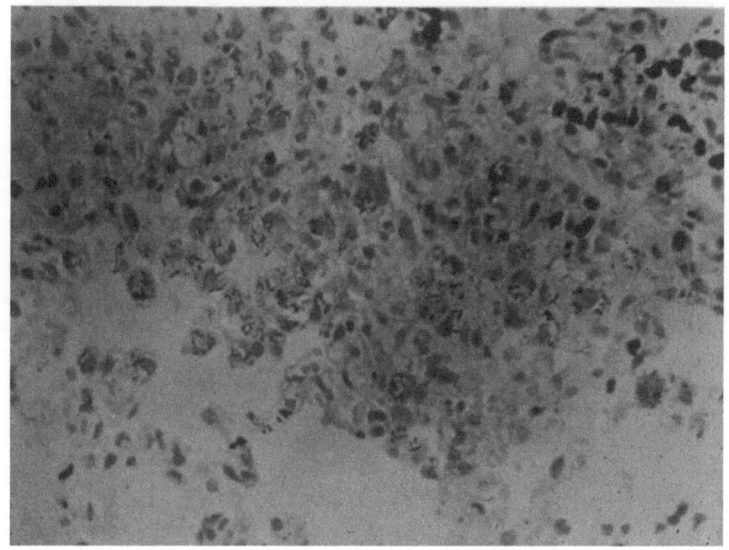

FIGURE 5. PRIMITIVE LESION IN A CORTISONE-TREATED RABBIT TWO WEEKS AFTER THE SAME INHALATION AS IN FIGURE 3, INDICATING MARKED INTRACELLULAR MULTIPLICATION OF BACILLI DUE TO CORTISONE TREATMENT

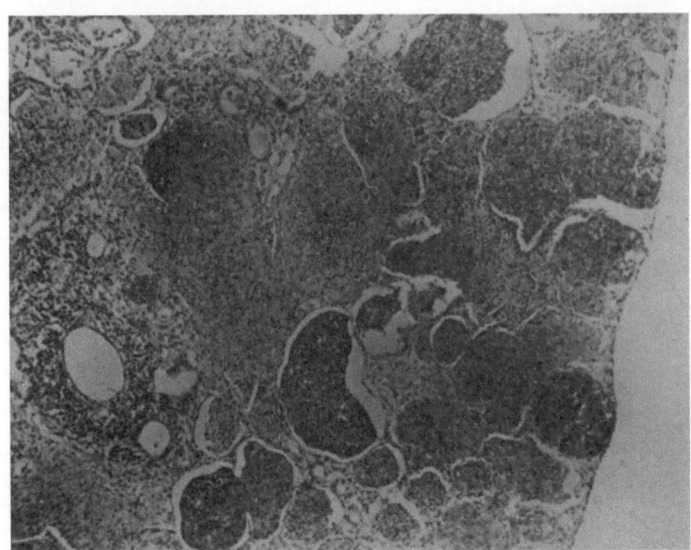

FIGURE 6. THE LESION IN THE LUNG OF A CORTISONE-TREATED RABBIT FIVE WEEKS AFTER INHALATION INFECTION, REVEALING PARTIALLY CASEATED PNEUMONIC PLUGS IN THE ALVEOLI AND LITTLE INFLAMMATION IN THE ALVEOLAR SEPTA ABOUT THEM

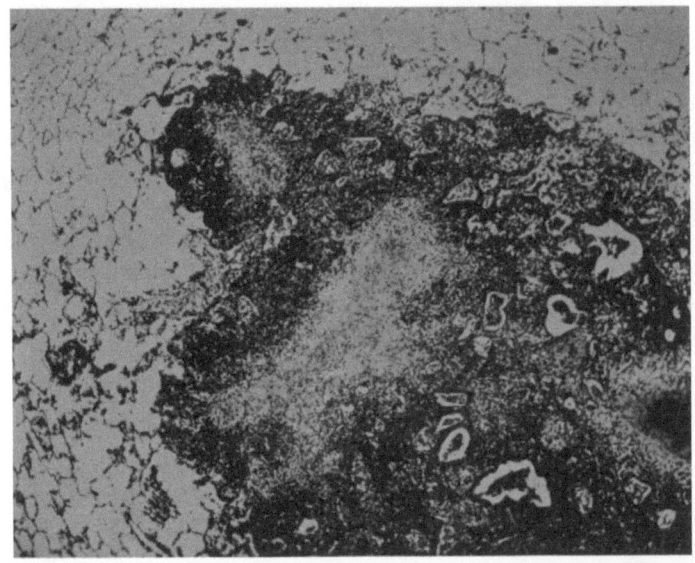

FIGURE 7. THE LESION IN THE LUNG OF AN UNTREATED RABBIT FIVE WEEKS AFTER THE SAME INHALATION AS IN FIGURE 6, INDICATING MATURE CASEATION AND EXTENSIVE PERIFOCAL INFLAMMATION

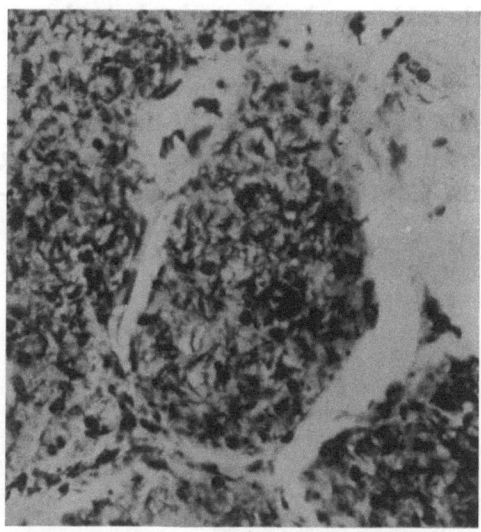

FIGURE 8. INORDINATE ACCUMULATION OF HUMAN TYPE TUBERCLE BACILLI IN THE PARTIALLY CASEATED ALVEOLAR PLUGS OF THE CORTISONE-TREATED RABBIT

inflammation, penetrated by ingrowing capillaries (Fig. 6). Hence, though the bacilli in the pulmonary lesions of the untreated animals were by far fewer than in the experimental rabbits, invasion of the blood and lymph by the bacilli occurred in the former, but not in the latter.

Much of the difference in the pathogenesis of tuberculosis in the two types of animals may be understood on the basis of the observed protection afforded the capillaries by cortisone against agents, prevalent in tuberculous lesions, which increase capillary permeability. This explains not only the suppression of the perifocal inflammation about the intraalveolar plugs swarming with tubercle bacilli in the cortisone-treated rabbits but also the marked reduction of the tuberculin reaction in these rabbits. Withdrawal of cortisone reverts the sensitivity of the capillary walls to agents which increase permeability to its original state and the consequent intensification of the tuberculin reaction and the development of an intense perifocal inflammation about the accumulated masses of bacilli in the lungs which resulted from the previous hormone treatment. This leads to massive pulmonary tuberculosis, with liquefaction, rupture into the bronchi, hematogenous dissemination, and death of naturally susceptible rabbits and to progressive disease with cavity formation in naturally resistant rabbits (Figs. 9–10). At the same time the lesions in the simultaneously infected untreated rabbits regress rapidly in the susceptible rabbits or heal completely in the resistant animals.

No evidence has thus far been obtained to indicate that the inordinate accumulation of the tubercle bacilli in the cells of the cortisone-treated rabbits may be accounted for by the hormone's stimulating effect on the growth of the bacilli. Cortisone, in the concentration pres-

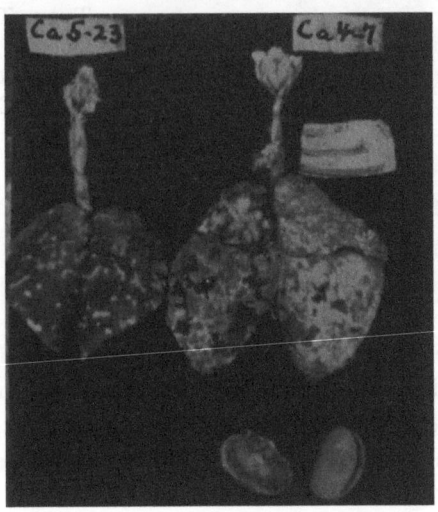

FIGURE 9. THE LUNGS OF A NATIVELY SUSCEPTIBLE RABBIT (Ca 5-23), AN UNTREATED CONTROL, AND A CORTISONE-TREATED RABBIT (Ca 4-7)

October 12, 1950 both animals inhaled an estimated 26,000 and 16,000 tubercle bacilli respectively. Ca 4-7 was under cortisone treatment from October 8, 1950, to November 22, 1950. It died thirty-four days after withdrawal of the hormone, of massive caseous pneumonia, liquefaction, rupture into the bronchi, and hematogenous dissemination. Ca 5-23 was killed one day later. The lungs show regressive tubercles with evidence of healing.

ent in the body of the experimental animals, does not enhance the growth of tubercle bacilli in vitro. The extracellular multiplication of the bacilli in vivo was markedly suppressed when bacilli within collodion-coated silk bags were placed into the peritoneal cavity of hormone-treated rabbits. That cortisone fundamentally affects the physiology of macrophages is evident from the enhanced phagocytic capacity afforded them by the hormone; yet the digestive capacity of these cells for tubercle bacilli is markedly depressed.

Summary.—Cortisone affects the essential mechanisms involved in the pathogenesis of tuberculosis. It increases the accumulation of tubercle bacilli within the macrophages, despite their enhanced phagocytic activity. It suppresses nonspecific and allergic inflammation, possibly as a result of the protective effect exerted by the hormone against many agents which increase capillary permeability. This antiphlogistic influence, by suppressing the ingrowth of capillaries into the tubercles and thus interrupting the bridge between the focus and the rest of the body, may be responsible for partial isolation of the lesion and for its

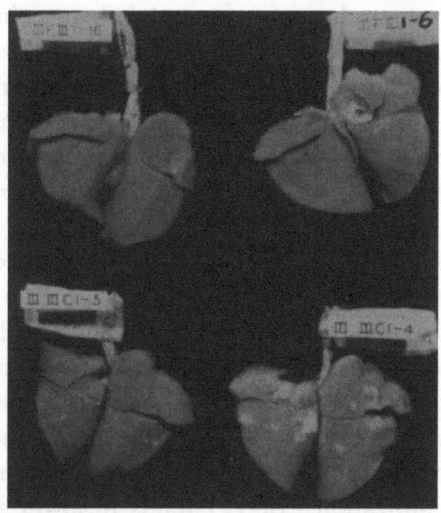

FIGURE 10. THE LUNGS OF GENETICALLY RESISTANT RABBIT IIIFIII 1-16, AN UNTREATED CONTROL, AND IIIFIII 1-6, A CORTISONE-TREATED RABBIT

February 21, 1951 both inhaled 2,800 and 3,100 human type tubercle bacilli, H37Rv, respectively. IIIFIII 1-6 was under cortisone treatment from February 12, 1951, to April 20, 1951. The rabbit was killed 28 days after withdrawal of the hormone. Two large thick walled cavities were found in the right lung, one of which can be seen in the photograph. IIIFIII 1-16 was killed on May 21, 1951. A slight regressive residual tubercle was found in the lower lobe of the left lung.

THE LUNGS OF THE GENETICALLY RESISTANT RABBITS III IIIC 1-5, AN UNTREATED CONTROL, AND III IIIC 1-4, A CORTISONE-TREATED RABBIT. February 21, 1951, both inhaled about 2,400 and 3,300 human type tubercle bacilli, H37Rv. III IIIC 1-4 was under cortisone treatment from February 12, 1951, to April 20, 1951. It was killed May 21, 1951. There was extensive tuberculosis in both lungs. III IIIC 1-5, killed on the same day, showed a few minute regressing tubercles in the lungs.

temporary and partial localization at the portal of entry. The reduced capillary permeability and the lympholytic effect of the hormone may also be instrumental in retarding the development of the caseous process and diminishing the antibody production which is characteristic of the cortisone-treated animals. Studies directed to elucidate the effect of cortisone on the intercellular ground substance, on cellular permeability, and on the enzyme functions of the phagocytes are in progress. Beside these specific effects of pharmacologic doses of cortisone on the disease, the hormone produces fundamental changes in the entire economy of the body. Among them are the marked atrophy of the fascicular and reticular zones of the adrenal, the great enlargement of the liver cells by excessive storage of glycogen and fat, and the atrophy of the spleen, thyroid, and male gonads. How each of these conspicuous metabolic effects influence the pathogenesis of the disease remains to be determined.

Thus, in tuberculosis cortisone acts like a double-edged sword. The very suppression of the inflammation, while it tends to isolate the infection from the rest of the body, nevertheless permits the local multiplication of the bacteria. For the phagocytes and the humoral agents concerned with combating the infection arrive tardily and in low concentration. Furthermore, there is general agreement, including observations presented in this symposium, that cortisone administered during the course of immunization (10–11) tends to lower antibody production, which would also militate against the infected host. Again, while there is ample evidence that increased adrenal function and cortisone stimulate phagocytosis of particulate matter and bacteria (12), the digestive capacity of the cells for the ingested microorganisms is markedly reduced, whether they be tubercle bacilli, pneumococci (13), streptococci (14), or even red blood cells (15). Hence the bacteria can accumulate in the tissues in the absence of symptoms of fever and toxemia which are suppressed by the hormone (16). However, it is possible that physiologic rather than pharmacologic doses of these and other adrenocortical and hypophyseal hormones may actually enhance the defense mechanisms against infection; but this remains to be determined.

REFERENCES

1. Lurie, M. B., and others, Constitutional factors in resistance to infection, *Am. Rev. Tuberc.*, 1949, 59:168, 186, 198.

2. Lurie, M. B., Mechanisms affecting spread in tuberculosis, *Ann. N.Y. Acad. Sci.*, 1950, 52:1074.
3. Lurie, M. B., S. Abramson, and A. G. Heppleston, Varying genetic resistance of rabbits to quantitative inhalation of human tubercle bacilli, *Fed. Proc.*, 1949, 8:361.
4. Lurie, M. B., The use of the rabbit in experimental chemotherapy of tuberculosis, *Ann. N.Y. Acad. Sci.*, 1949, 52:627.
   Lurie, M. B., S. Abramson, and A. G. Heppleston, On the response of genetically susceptible and resistant rabbits to the quantitative inhalation of human type tubercle bacilli and the nature of resistance to tuberculosis, *J. Exp. Med.*, 1952, 95:119.
5. Lurie, M. B., A. G. Heppleston, S. Abramson and I. B. Swartz, An evaluation of the method of quantitative airborne infection and its use in the study of the pathogenesis of tuberculosis, *Am. Rev. Tuberc.*, 1950, 61:765.
6. Menkin, V., Further studies on effect of adrenal cortex extract and of various steroids on capillary permeability, *Proc. Soc. Exp. Biol. & Med.*, 1942, 51:39.
7. Ungar, G., and E. Damgaard, Studies on the fibrinolysin-antifibrinolysin system of serums; I: Action of pituitary, adrenal cortex and spleen, *J. Exp. Med.*, 1951, 93:89.
8. Middlebrook, G., and R. J. Dubos, Specific serum agglutination of erythrocytes sensitized with extracts of tubercle bacilli, *J. Exp. Med.*, 1948, 88:521.
9. Gordon, A. S., and G. Katsh, The relation of the adrenal cortex to the structure and phagocytic activity of the macrophagic system, *Ann. N.Y. Acad. Sci.*, 1949, 52:1.
10. Germuth, F. G., J. Oyama, and B. Ottinger, The mechanism of action of 17-hydroxy-11-dehydrocorticosterone (compound E) and of the adrenocorticotrophic hormone in experimental hypersensitivity in rabbits, *J. Exp. Med.*, 1951, 94:139.
11. Fischel, E. E., Adrenal hormones and the development of antibody and hypersensitivity. This symposium, chapter 6.
12. Kuna, A., B. Blattberg, and J. Reiman, Effect of starvation on phagocytosis in vivo, *Proc. Soc. Exp. Biol. & Med.*, 1951, 77:510.
13. Robinson, H. J., Effect of cortisone on intradermal pneumococcal infections in rabbits, *Fed. Proc.*, 1951, 10:332.
14. Thomas, L., The effect of cortisone and ACTH on the response of animals to certain bacteria and bacterial toxins. This symposium, chapter 12.
15. Kass, E. H., Q. M. Geiman, and M. Finland, Observations on adrenal cortical hormones in pneumococcal and influenza viral infections and in malaria. This symposium, chapter 13.
16. Dubois-Ferriere, H., Risk of infection associated with prolonged treatment with adrenocorticotrophic hormone (ACTH) and cortisone, *Praxis*, 1950, 39:974.

Chapter 9

STUDIES ON THE MECHANISM OF ACTION OF CORTISONE IN EXPERIMENTAL SYPHILIS [1]

By THOMAS B. TURNER AND DAVID H. HOLLANDER, *Department of Microbiology, The Johns Hopkins University School of Hygiene and Public Health*

THERE IS ABUNDANT EVIDENCE indicating that profound changes are initiated in the human and animal hosts by an abnormal amount of adrenal cortical hormone, supplied either directly in the form of cortisone or compound F or indirectly by stimulating the adrenal cortex by other hormonal substances, such as adrenocorticotrophic hormone (ACTH). That these agents bring about significant alteration in the response of a host to infectious agents is becoming increasingly clear, but the mechanisms by which these effects are induced are still obscure.

As a biological system for the study of some of these effects experimental syphilis offers certain attractive features, for the evolution of the disease proceeds step-wise in an orderly fashion; discrete syphilitic lesions of considerable uniformity can be produced in the skin, where they can be readily observed; some of the important factors influencing the evolution of these lesions are known; and the infection can be terminated within a period of hours by penicillin without immediately altering the tissue response substantially. The following paper, which is an extension of a preliminary report (1), is concerned primarily with consideration of the basic mechanisms of action of cortisone in this experimental infection.

THE USUAL COURSE OF EXPERIMENTAL SYPHILIS

The incubation period of syphilitic lesions following intradermal inoculation is largely a function of the number of *Treponema pallidum* injected. Under optimum conditions it is approximately ten to twenty days when five hundred organisms are inoculated into each site, and it

[1] Aided by grants from the National Institutes of Health, Bethesda, Maryland, and the Whitehall Foundation, New York.

varies from about thirty days with a small inoculum to three to four days when the inoculum contains in the order of five million treponemes. Experimental evidence indicates that for each ten-fold decrease in the number of treponemes the incubation period is prolonged by about four days (2–4). The multiplication of treponemes at the site of inoculation seems to proceed logarithmically after the first twenty-four or forty-eight hours, so that a division time of approximately thirty hours can be deduced. Substantial variations of the incubation periods from the theoretical values rarely occur. One of the principle causes of variation, excluding counting difficulties, is probably temperature; summer temperatures, for example, being known to have a definite suppressing effect on the development of lesions. In the present experiments animals were kept in air-conditioned rooms at a temperature of approximately 20°C (68°F) or somewhat lower.

A group of rabbits in a uniform environment will respond to a given inoculum in a remarkably uniform manner. One-tenth ml. of material is customarily inoculated intradermally into each of four, six, or eight sites on the clipped back of the rabbit. With few exceptions, rabbits inoculated with the same batch of material develop a characteristic pattern of tiny lesions within twenty-four hours of each other, and almost without exception the lesions in the same animal appear simultaneously and go through successive stages of evolution together. Testicular lesions induced by direct inoculation follow essentially the same pattern, although the incubation periods are usually somewhat longer, at least partly because the early reaction cannot be visualized, but must be recognized by palpation.

Once cutaneous papules have developed at the sites of inoculation they increase rapidly in size and reach a maximum in about a week. At this stage the lesion has a characteristic appearance, being elevated, with a flat surface and a sharply circumscribed circular base, which often measures 10–15 mm in diameter. The lesions are dusky red and are invariably firm or hard in consistency. In fixed and stained preparations the lesions show a characteristic mononuclear infiltration which typically tends to have a perivascular distribution. In addition there is usually an accumulation of a mucinous material, which does not stain with hematoxylin or eosin. This substance has been tentatively identified as hyaluronic acid by Scott and Dammin (5), and our findings support this conclusion.

When the well-developed syphiloma is incised, fluid material is exuded freely from the cut surface. The fluid may be slightly stringy because of the presence of a small or moderate amount of the mucoid material. This fluid contains actively motile *T. pallidum* in abundance, and a rough approximation of the relative numbers of treponemes in the lesion can be made by the use of appropriate counting techniques (6). About 0.05 ml. of fluid is collected on a coverslip, and the count is expressed as the number of treponemes present per 100 oil-immersion fields, the counts being made on the same darkfield microscope or one with approximately the same calibration. Ordinarily counts are made on two lesions of the same animal, and the two counts are expressed as a mean value. While this method of counting is obviously far from precise, it yields reasonably repeatable results.

Within a week after the syphiloma has reached its maximum size, the surface of the lesion undergoes necrosis (Fig. 1), and eventually the entire lesion may be covered with an adherent scab. Thereafter resolution takes place; the lesions often disappear within another two weeks, although at times the healing period is protracted. There is a relationship in the time of the healing process to the time of the development of immunity to challenge inoculation and the rise in titer of immobilizing antibody (7).

Generalized lesions of the skin and bones occasionally occur, but they seem to be less frequent following intracutaneous than intratesticular inoculation, and much less common than after intravenous inoculation (8).

Within two months after the appearance of symptoms the animal usually has no recognizable syphilitic lesions. The lymph nodes, however, remain infectious for normal rabbits, although treponemes are not sufficiently numerous to be seen on darkfield examination.[2]

The foregoing brief sketch of the evolution of experimental syphilis in the rabbit is based on the observation of a good many hundreds of animals and provides a background of experience for the evaluation of both the test and control animals used in the present experiments.

The effect of cortisone on the evolution of experimental syphilis.—

---

[2] With the ordinary darkfield oil-immersion microscope material containing 100,000 spirochetes per ml. will show on the average 1 treponeme in about 50 fields; when the count falls much below this only rarely is it possible to demonstrate treponemes by the darkfield microscope.

EXPERIMENTAL SYPHILIS

Cortisone[3] was given in the form of a saline suspension of cortisone acetate (Cortone-Merck), the usual dose being 3.0 mg per kilogram body weight of the animal, administered intramuscularly twice daily, commonly at about 9 A.M. and 5:30 P.M. In some experiments smaller doses were given or administration was limited to once daily. The duration of treatment varied from five days in some experiments to more than sixty days in others.

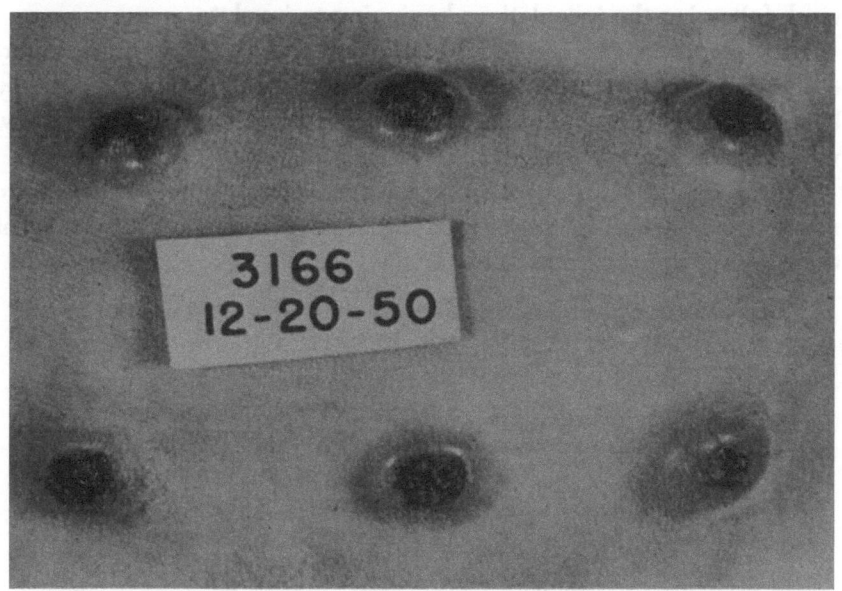

FIGURE 1. BACK LESIONS OF RABBIT 3166 (EXP. 77E, GROUP D) Each site inoculated with 50,000 T. *pallidum* on 11/24/50. Typical pattern appeared on 9th day; ulceration first noted on 24th day; photographed on 26th day. Height of numerals approximately 4.4 mm.

The Nichols strain of *T. pallidum* was used throughout, and animals were usually observed daily. In most experiments the lesions were measured, drawn, and photographed at intervals. Altogether 143 rabbits are included in the experiments reported here, of which 91 had been given cortisone at one time or another, and 52 served as controls.

Effect on well-developed syphilomas.—In the initial experiment (Exp. 77A) six rabbits were inoculated intradermally at each of four

[3] Most of the cortisone used in these experiments was supplied without cost by Merck and Company.

sites with 500 *T. pallidum*. On the twenty-fifth day after inoculation, when the lesions in all animals were approaching their maximum size, three animals were given cortisone, three mg per kilogram intramuscularly twice daily for a total of ten doses, and three animals were kept as untreated controls.

The lesions in the control animals evolved in the expected manner (Fig. 1), becoming somewhat larger, then ulcerating, and within one week following the inoculations beginning to involute.

The lesions in the cortisone-treated animals behaved quite differently. Beginning with the second day of cortisone administration, they became globoid in configuration, pale in color, and soft and spongy, with a sharply circumscribed base (Fig. 2).

On the day of the last cortisone injection counts of treponeme were made in one lesion in the treated and control rabbits. The results of these counts are shown in Table 1.

TREPONEME COUNTS ON SYPHILOMAS OF CORTISONE-TREATED AND CONTROL RABBITS

GROUP	RABBIT NUMBER	DARKFIELD TREPONEME COUNTS NUMBER PER 100 OIL-IMMERSION FIELDS POST-TREATMENT DAY		
		Fifth	Seventh	Tenth
Cortisone treated [a]	29–63	3,000	2,960	2,300
	29–66	1,500	1,002	680
	29–67	750	406	1,650
Controls	29–62	116	27	7
	29–64	140	69	156
	29–65	224	35	3

[a] Inoculated with 500 *T. pallidum* in Each of Four Sites; cortisone 3 mgm/kg twice daily for 10 doses started 25th day after inoculation.

It is evident that there is a striking difference between the number of *T. pallidum* in the cortisone-treated animals and the controls. By the time the first counts were made, that is, five days after beginning the cortisone injections, the lesions in the control animals had begun to subside and the counts obtained on those lesions were as had been expected from previous experience. On the other hand, the counts in one of the cortisone-treated animals were much higher than had ever been encountered.[4] Actually the figures given for these counts are probably too

[4] For other comparative data see Reference 6; note that counts in that paper are expressed in numbers per 200 fields.

low, for the treponemes were swarming over the entire field, rendering accurate counts impossible.

Two days after cessation of cortisone treatment it was noted that the lesions in the treated animals had begun to increase in size, and within another twenty-four hours they had become enlarged to enormous proportions, were tense, erythematous, and showed considerable new in-

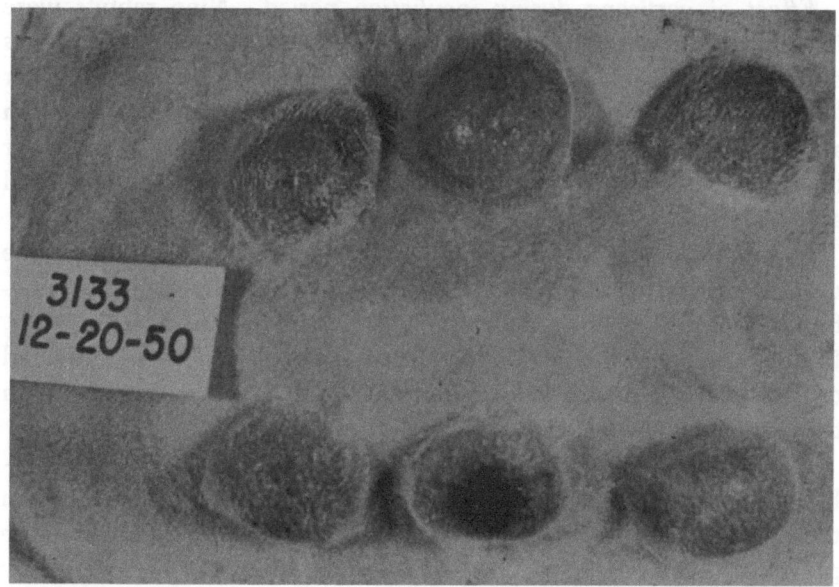

FIGURE 2. BACK LESIONS OF RABBIT 3133 (EXP. 77E, GROUP A) Inoculated as was rabbit 3166. Typical pattern appeared on 9th day; cortisone 3 mgm/kg twice daily given for 2 weeks, beginning 12th day; photographed at time of last treatment on 26th day. Note large globoid appearance and absence of ulceration.

filtration spreading out from the base of the lesion. We have designated this the "rebound." Counts at this time and again three days later were still high (Table 1). After one to two weeks the lesions, too, began to subside slowly.

It was mentioned in the preceding section that for a few days at the height of their evolution syphilomas frequently contain small or moderate amounts of a mucinous material. In this experiment the lesions in the control animals had passed the point at which this material is usually present to any considerable extent. In striking contrast, however, the lesions of the cortisone-treated rabbits appeared to be filled with this gelatinous-like material, so that it oozed from the cut surface in greater abundance than has ever been observed by us except in cortisone-treated rabbits.

This experiment has been repeated, with some variation, in sixty additional animals, forty-two cortisone-treated, and eighteen controls, with essentially the same results.

Effect of cortisone during incubation period.—Nine rabbits were inoculated intradermally with 1,000,000 *T. pallidum* at each of six sites on the clipped back (Exp. 77C). In three rabbits cortisone, 3 mg per kilogram twice daily, was begun twenty-four hours prior to inoculation and continued for six days or until within approximately twenty-four hours of the expected time of appearance of lesions in the untreated animals.

In another group of three rabbits in this series cortisone in the same dosage was started approximately twenty-four to forty-eight hours before lesions developed in the controls, and was continued for five days. In this experiment the incubation period of the lesions in the untreated controls was five days in one and six days in two, as was expected with this size inoculum.

In the group receiving cortisone before and during most of the incubation period, lesions appeared on the sixth day, approximately as in the controls, but they progressed more slowly and resembled those previously observed under cortisone therapy. These changes were only temporary, however, for within a few days the lesions took on the characteristics of those in the untreated controls.

In the group of three rabbits in which cortisone was started twenty-four to forty-eight hours before the expected appearance of lesions, the incubation period was essentially unmodified, being six days in two, and seven days in one. In each animal the evolution of the lesions was at a considerably slower pace than in the controls, and by the end of the course of cortisone therapy (on the ninth day) the difference was marked, the lesions being much smaller than in the controls and presenting the characteristic appearance of those in rabbits treated with cortisone. Within two to three days after cortisone was discontinued the typical "rebound" phenomenon was noted.

Effect on subsiding lesions.—In four rabbits cortisone 3 mg/kg was given when lesions had been present for twenty-four days and were still active, but were apparently beginning to subside. In each a typical cortisone effect, followed by a rebound, was noted.

In another group of five rabbits cortisone 3.0 mg/kg was given once daily for five days, beginning approximately fifty to sixty days after cutaneous syphilomas had first appeared, when the healing stage was well advanced. No modification in the size or character of the lesions were noted either during or subsequent to cortisone therapy.

These results suggest that once the immune mechanism has come fully into play, reactivation of lesions is not readily accomplished by short courses of cortisone. The experiments, however, are inadequate to show conclusively that a latent syphilitic infection cannot be reactivated by cortisone.

Effect of long-continued cortisone therapy.—In a group of fourteen rabbits (Exp. 77D) inoculated with 500 *T. pallidum* at each of six sites, seven animals were treated with cortisone 3 mg/kg once daily for twenty-eight doses, beginning within two days after lesions appeared, and seven animals were maintained as controls. All the treated animals developed typical globoid, soft, pale lesions (Fig. 2), which differed strikingly from those in the controls (Fig. 1). Most of the treated animals lost weight, but whether this was due to the direct effects of the cortisone, to the syphilitic infection, or to intercurrent infection was not definitely ascertained.

Upon withdrawal of cortisone all of the six surviving animals exhibited the rebound phenomenon, and five developed generalized lesions of the skin, one of them to an extent never previously observed. Only two of the seven control animals developed generalized syphilitic papules, and these only sparsely. Three of the treated animals developed subcutaneous abscesses which were obviously nonsyphilitic.

White blood-cell counts and blood-serological tests were made at intervals on the animals in this experiment; the results will be discussed later.

In a similar experiment (Exp. 77E) five groups of eight rabbits each were inoculated intracutaneously with 50,000 *T. pallidum* in each of six sites on the clipped back. Lesions appeared in all about the tenth day. Beginning on the thirteenth day after inoculation, the animals were treated with cortisone, as follows:

Group A—3mg/kg twice daily for 2 weeks; Group B—3 mg/kg twice daily for 4 weeks; Group C—1 mg/kg once daily for 2 weeks; Group D—1 mg/kg once daily for 4 weeks; and Group E (controls)—no cortisone.

At intervals the lesions of one animal from each group were excised for histological study. White-blood counts were made, and blood was taken for serological tests on surviving animals at fortnightly intervals.

Consideration for the moment will be limited to the "large-dose" groups and the controls (Group A, B, and E). Within two to four days after the first injection of cortisone all treated animals developed lesions of characteristic configuration and appearance and were in striking contrast to those which had received no cortisone.

In Group A all eight animals survived the two-week treatment period, lesions from two being taken on the last day of treatment. Of the remaining six, all developed typical and rather violent rebound reactions, five within three to seven days after the last treatment, but one not until twenty-one days after the final treatment. In the latter animal there may have been a depot of cortisone which was not entirely depleted for several weeks.

The rebound followed the usual pattern insofar as the cutaneous syphilomas were concerned. The lesions enlarged rapidly, became much more indurated, and often satellite papules appeared in the clipped area. In addition several animals developed extensive cutaneous and subcutaneous abscesses, in which organisms of the *Pasteurella* group appeared to be playing the principal etiological role. Two animals died during this period, presumably of *Pasteurella* infection, and there was little doubt that the cortisone had likewise substantially altered the host-parasite relationship to the disadvantage of the host with regard to this group of organisms, as well as to the induced syphilitic infection.

Lesions from one animal of this group were excised on the seventh post-treatment day; in the three surviving animals the syphilitic lesions, after going through the characteristic rebound, began to retrogress two to three weeks after the last treatment.

Among Group B animals, those which received cortisone over a four-week period, one died early in the course of treatment, but the other seven developed syphilitic lesions of the type characteristically observed with cortisone therapy, globoid, pale, soft, and sharply delineated as compared with the rather flat, hard, broad-based lesions so characteristically seen in the controls.

During the third and fourth weeks of cortisone therapy the response of the animals varied considerably, but in most an apparent "escape" from the effects of cortisone was noted in that either the rebound began or healing began while the animal was still under therapy. Of the seven rabbits in this group, one died after nineteen days of cortisone therapy, when the lesions were beginning to revert to the "control" type, and another, which had shown typical cortisone type lesions throughout, was sacrificed for histological study on the last day of therapy. In two animals healing began during the last two weeks of treatment without an obvious rebound; in three animals a rebound began during the last two weeks of treatment which resulted in the development of enormous lesions, with extensive generalized lesions in one.

It should be noted that this "escape" phenomenon was not observed in the animals of Group A, which received treatment for fourteen days. It would seem from this experiment that upon prolonged cortisone therapy a degree of tolerance to the drug may develop.

The effect of smaller doses of cortisone.—In one of the earlier experiments three rabbits with well-developed dermal syphilomas were given cortisone twice daily in doses of 1.5 mg per kilogram instead of 3.0 mg/kg. With this smaller dose essentially the same changes were noted as with the larger dose.

Included in the experiment (77E) of the preceding section was one group of rabbits (Group C) which was given 1.0 mg per kilogram once daily for two weeks and a group (Group D) which was given the same dose for four weeks. In other words, Groups C and D received one-sixth the dose of Groups A and B, respectively.

Of the sixteen rabbits in the two groups, all developed lesions which were fairly characteristic of those observed with larger doses of cortisone. During the second week of cortisone therapy the lesions in many animals began to "escape," as it were, from the influence of cortisone and became more indurated. Among the animals in which cortisone was discontinued after fourteen days of therapy, lesions were taken from one on the fourteenth day. The remaining seven developed a fairly characteristic rebound phenomenon, the lesions increasing rapidly in size and becoming indurated and rather flat in configuration, as were those of the controls.

Among the animals in Group D, in which daily treatment was continued for twenty-eight days, lesions from one were excised for histological study at the end of treatment; the remaining seven developed during therapy a type of lesion showing characteristics that partook of those in both the control animals and in animals receiving larger doses of cortisone. These lesions were large, of rubbery consistence, and very rich in spirochetes.

Effect on testicular lesions.—*T. pallidum* inoculated into the rabbit's testis invokes after an appropriate incubation period the development of an orchitis characterized by enlargement, and induration. Cortisone induced essentially the same changes in these lesions as was noted in the cutaneous syphilomas, and the testes were filled with mucoid material containing enormous numbers of spirochetes. It has been shown in this laboratory that cortisone-treated animals afford a rich source of *T. pallidum* for the treponemal immobilization test; these findings having been confirmed by DeLamater, Saurino, and Urbach (9).

Nature of the mucoid material.—The occurrence of metachromatic staining material in experimentally induced syphilomas in rabbits has been previously noted by Scott and Dammin (5), as well as by earlier workers. In our animals treated with cortisone this material accumulated in great abundance and was of a stringy and tenacious mucoid consistency. Exposure of this material, either in vivo or in vitro, to hyaluronidase prepared from bull's testes, resulted in its prompt transformation to a thin, fluid consistency. Motile treponemes were still abundant in this material.

In formalin fixed-tissue sections the mucoid material is stained purple by toluidene blue, but if the section is first treated with bull testis hyaluronidase the metachromatic staining property is completely eliminated and the mucoid areas remain unstained.

Using the methods of Pearce and Watson (10), our associate Dr. Frederick Rice has analyzed cortisone-treated and nontreated syphilomas for hyaluronic acid and chondroitin sulfate. From the lesions of the cortisone-treated animals a large amount was recovered as hyaluronic acid, and very little as chondroitin sulfate, while from the nontreated lesions very little hyaluronic acid, but a large amount of the chondroitin sulfate fraction, was obtained. Clinical determinations for glucosamine, nitrogen, sulfate, and water gave values which were consistent with the values reported for hyaluronic acid and chondroitin sulfate (11–13). The hyaluronic acid fraction from syphilomas analysed as follows: hexosamine 28.4 percent, sulfate 0.0 percent, nitrogen 3.3 percent. Values for the chondroitin sulfate fraction were: hexosamine 25.5 percent, sulfate 12.5 percent, and nitrogen 1.48 percent.

An attempt was made to determine quantitatively the hyaluronic acid

EXPERIMENTAL SYPHILIS

and chondroitin sulfate content in a series of lesions from treated and untreated animals. However, apparently the available methods are not sufficiently sensitive to provide reliable comparative data.

The foregoing histologic, enzymatic, and chemical evidence indicates that the mucoid material is hyaluronic acid and suggests that a prominent component of the untreated syphiloma is a chondroitin-like material. One is led to speculate concerning the source of this abundant hyaluronic acid. Beyond question its formation in such large amounts results directly or indirectly from the presence of *T. pallidum*. Whether the material stems directly from the treponemes itself or is a product of the tissue reaction invoked by the treponeme has not been conclusively determined, but it seems likely that the former supposition is correct. It is further suggested that the indurated character of the usual syphilomas, as well as the rebound lesions, may be due to the conversion of the treponemal hyaluronic acid to a sulfated molecule of the nature of chondroitin sulfate.

Histopathological changes induced by cortisone.—Early in the evolution of cutaneous syphilomas the lesions are characterized by the accumulation of an intracellular mucoid material which has been identified as hyaluronic acid, and a marked infiltration of mononuclear cells with a typical perivascular distribution (Fig. 3). As the evolution of the lesions proceeds, phagocytic cells and fibroblasts appear. When ulceration supervenes there is extensive nonspecific necrosis, with large numbers of polymorphonuclear cells.

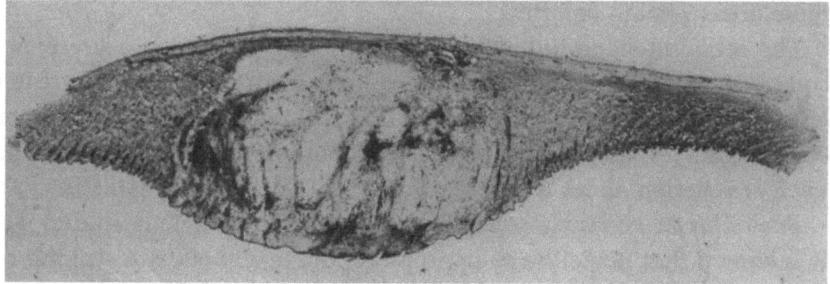

FIGURE 3. LESION FROM RABBIT 3172 (EXP. 77E, GROUP D)
Inoculated as was rabbit 3166. Typical pattern appeared on 9th day; no cortisone given; section taken on 26th day at the early stage of ulceration. Note darkly staining areas of cellular infiltrate as well as unstained areas of mucoid material (Hematoxylin and eosin).

In the lesions of animals treated with cortisone there is a marked increase in the amount of hyaluronic acid (Fig. 4), and as mentioned previously treponemes are also present in much greater numbers than in animals receiving no cortisone. At the same time cellular infiltration is almost entirely lacking, so that the main mass of the lesion appears to be composed entirely of hyaluronic acid. Necrosis is not present in the typical cortisone lesions.

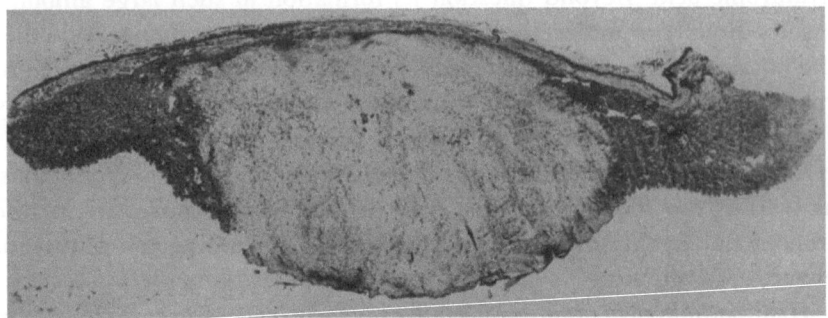

FIGURE 4. LESION FROM RABBIT 3137 (EXP. 77E, GROUP A)
Inoculated as was rabbit 3166. Typical pattern appeared on 9th day; cortisone 3 mgm/kg twice daily given for 2 weeks beginning on 12th day; section taken on 26th day; no ulceration. Note large amount of nonstaining mucoid material and almost complete absence of cellular infiltrate.

The hyaluronic acid in formalin-fixed sections stains distinctly purple with toluidine blue, but when pretreated with bull testis hyaluronidase these areas remain colorless.

The rebound stage following the withdrawal of cortisone presents a complicated picture which resembles various aspects of the untreated lesions. There are rapid accumulations of mononuclear cells and numerous phagocytes, as well as fibroblastic proliferation and a polymorphonuclear reaction about a central ulcer.

Penicillin in cortisone-treated animals.—From previous studies (6) it is known that penicillin in appropriate doses will effect a striking reduction in the treponeme count of cutaneous syphilomas in rabbits within twenty-four hours. Employing a previously outlined approach, six cortisone-treated rabbits and two controls were given penicillin, and treponeme counts were made on the lesions before and twenty-four hours after the initial dose of penicillin. At the time penicillin was administered, three of the test animals had received cortisone for four days, and three for seven days; in each the cutaneous syphilomas showed the typical changes induced by cortisone. The prepenicillin treponeme counts were very high. In the control animals the lesions were similar to those ordinarily seen in rabbits in the absence of cortisone, and the prepenicillin counts were substantially lower. All animals received a total dose of 5 mg crystalline penicillin G per kg intramuscularly in aqueous solution divided into three equal doses at two-hour intervals.

Treponeme counts on the lesions twenty-four hours after the initial dose of penicillin showed a marked reduction in the number of motile treponemes in all animals. As customarily observed, in the control animals only an occasional treponeme, either motile or nonmotile, was observed. In the lesions of the cortisone-treated animals an occasional motile treponeme and a larger number of nonmotile (and presumably dead) *T. pallidum* were observed in the darkfield preparations.

Although penicillin seems to be equally effective in killing treponemes in cortisone-treated and in non-cortisone-treated animals, the mechanism of clearing killed or damaged organisms from the lesions is apparently less efficient in the cortisone-treated animals; however the presence of larger numbers of nonmotile treponemes may merely be a reflection of the larger number of motile treponemes in the lesions before treatment.

Effect on serology.—In the five groups of animals referred to above (Exp. 77E), blood samples were taken before the administration of cortisone and at fortnightly intervals thereafter. Quantitative serologic tests for syphilis, employing cardiolipin antigen, were made on each sample, using both complement fixation and flocculation techniques. No clear-cut difference in pattern was observed among the five groups. In the groups of animals receiving the larger doses of cortisone the mean titer of so-called Wassermann antibody was slightly lower after two weeks of treatment than the mean titer in the groups receiving smaller doses or no treatment; but the differences were not remarkable, and there was considerable variation among individual animals. Routine tests for treponemal immobilization antibody was not made, because of technical difficulties in accurate quantitation. The few tests made indicated that cortisone did not cause any significant reduction in treponemal immobilization antibody.

Effect upon lymph nodes.—It is known that cortisone brings about a reduction in circulating lymphocytes and a generalized hypoplasia of lymphoid tissue (14). Since syphilis in the rabbit commonly causes pronounced hyperplasia of lymph nodes, it was of interest to observe the net effect of these two contrary forces.

The popliteal nodes of twelve cortisone-treated rabbits with active cutaneous syphilomas were found to be much smaller than in seven animals which had had no cortisone, and even smaller than those usually found in uninfected rabbits.

Effect upon circulating white blood cells. White-blood-cell counts were made on five groups of eight rabbits each, inoculated with *T. pallidum* at the same time and treated with different amounts of cortisone for varying lengths of time (See groups A, B, C, D, and E referred to above). In animals which had been treated with cortisone for twelve days the white counts were in general substantially lower than in the group which had received no cortisone, but little difference was noted between those receiving 3 mg/kg twice daily and those receiving 1 mg/kg once daily.

In animals treated for twenty-eight days the white counts were lower on the average than in the controls, but in these groups, as well as in those mentioned in the preceding paragraph, there were exceptions to the rule. At two and four weeks after the discontinuance of treatment the counts in the previously treated animals tended to be lower than in the controls.

Effect upon body weight.—The effect of cortisone on body weight is shown graphically in the diagram on p. 115. Animals receiving doses of cortisone in the order of 3 mg per kilogram consistently lost weight during treatment and for a week or two after treatment was discontinued. With doses approximately one-sixth of the large dose, weight loss occurred only after prolonged administration of cortisone. When cortisone was discontinued increase in body weight was customarily observed after a short interval.

Effect upon wound healing.—From the studies of Ragan and his associates (15) and others it is known that cortisone seriously interferes with wound healing, apparently because the treated animals fail to develop normal connective tissue cellular components, particularly fibroblasts. We have had opportunity to note in experiments in which syphilomas were excised for histological study that the operation

EXPERIMENTAL SYPHILIS

wounds healed less readily in those having received cortisone than in untreated animals.

Effect upon lipemia.—It has been previously reported by others that cortisone-treated animals show a marked increase in serum fats, large pale fatty livers, and atrophic spleens (14, 16–18). These changes were observed repeatedly in our animals which received as much as 3 mg/kg per day.

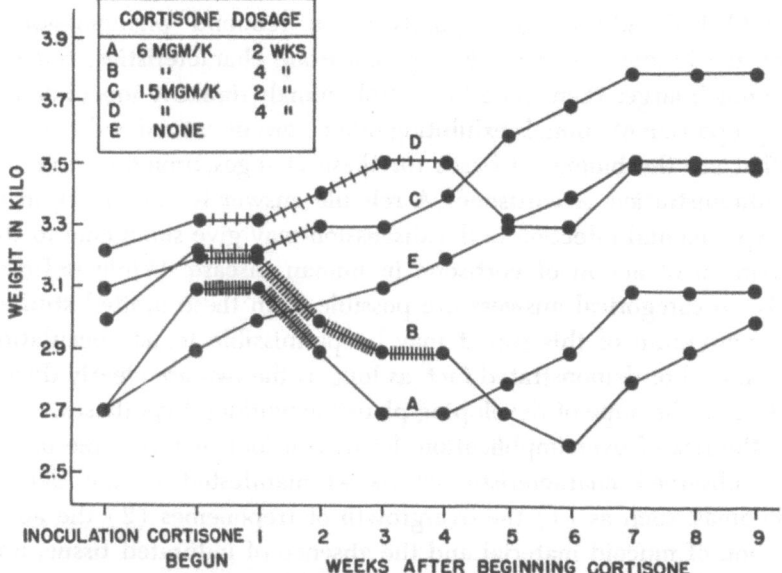

WEIGHT OF RABBITS DURING ADMINISTRATION OF CORTISONE

Discussion.—The administration of cortisone in moderate to large doses to rabbits with large dermal syphilomas induces remarkable changes in the lesions within a forty-eight hour period. These changes are characterized by transformation of the lesions from a cartilaginous consistency to a pale, soft, and sticky mucoid material identified as hyaluronic acid.

In the syphiloma of the untreated rabbit there is a marked mononuclear inflammatory reaction, with foci of *T. pallidum*. In the cortisone-treated animal the syphiloma is relatively acellular and the greatly increased mucoid material is swarming with actively motile *T. pallidum*.

At the height of the cortisone effect, although *T. pallidum* is present in the mucoid material in greater abundance than is ever observed in the absence of cortisone, the tissue response of the host is not at all characteristic of that commonly observed in syphilitic infection. In other words, the relationship between host and parasite has been abruptly altered, and the parasite flourishes without immediate reaction or damage to the host.

Upon withdrawal of cortisone, the normal relationships are quickly re-established and the host responds with a "rebound" phenomenon in which the lesions revert to their precortisone characteristics, but become much larger than those in control animals similarly inoculated, a high proportion of animals exhibiting other signs of extensive disease.

What are the biological bases for these changes brought about by the administration of cortisone? A reliable answer to this question in the experimental infection under discussion may give some clue to the mechanism of action of cortisone in human disease. While unfortunately no categorical answers are possible from these limited studies, in a symposium of this sort it may be permissible to let speculation range ahead of demonstrated fact, as long as the two are clearly distinguished, in the hope of developing plausible working hypotheses.

At the risk of oversimplification, let us consider merely three of the easily observed characteristic effects as manifested in the dermal syphilomas, such as (1) the overgrowth of treponemes (2) the accumulation of mucoid material and the absence of indurated tissue, and (3) the rebound upon the withdrawal of cortisone.

What are the important physiological effects promoting these changes? To consider first the overgrowth of treponemes in the lesions of cortisone-treated rabbits it should be recalled that under ordinary circumstances the evolution of the syphiloma is a process limited largely by the development of immunity, of which antibody formation is the humoral expression. The presence of excessive numbers of treponemes after cortisone treatment may conceivably be due either to suppression of this inhibiting antibody or to the creation of an environment unusually favorable to spirochetal survival and multiplication.

As brought out by other participants in the symposium, large doses of cortisone inhibit antibody formation. The doses employed in our experiments, however, were not as high as those used in most of the studies in which inhibition of antibody formation was demonstrated, and our results showed no consistent differences between groups of cortisone-treated rabbits and controls either in the pattern of Wassermann antibody or, less definitively, in the amount of treponemal immobilizing antibody.

Moreover, the changes in the lesions, both upon the administration of cortisone and upon its withdrawal, occurred so promptly that it is difficult to conceive that they could be attributed primarily to an effect on antibody titer. The presence of circulating antibody may not, however, be an accurate index of the amount of antibody available locally, and the marked reduction in cellular elements in the lesions of cortisone-treated animals may possibly result in decreased amounts of antibody at the site of the lesion.

On the other hand, the great accumulation of mucoid material in the lesion provides a physical environment which probably differs importantly from the usual one. There is experimental evidence suggesting that material of such mucoid consistency inhibits phagocytosis (19), and it may also offer a physical barrier to the diffusion of antibody, although there is no experimental evidence to support the latter suggestion.

The noteworthy effect of cortisone under these experimental conditions is the increase in the amount of mucoid material. Foci of actively multiplying *T. pallidum* in the rabbit are regularly associated with increased amounts of hyaluronic acid (5). The source of this mucoid material has not been definitely established. It is known that the normal ground substance of connective tissue contains small amounts of this material (20), but it seems more likely that the large amounts observed in syphilitic lesions in the rabbit are synthesized by the spirochete. Evidence is accumulating in our laboratory that species and strains of treponemes vary in their capacity to produce mucoid material and that this characteristic may be an important factor in determining the clinical picture of both the experimental and natural disease caused by these microorganisms.

This brings us to a consideration of another notable feature of the dermal syphilomas in cortisone-treated animals, namely, the replacement of cartilaginous-like tissue with this tenacious mucoid material. As mentioned above, the normal ground substance of connective tissue contains small amounts of hyaluronic acid, while certain other connective-tissue elements, such as tendons, cartilage, and other elastic tissue, contain chondroitin sulfate, a related mucopolysaccharide. There is some evidence, for example, that certain changes in skin, such as that observed in localized myxedema, are associated with an alteration in the ratio of hyaluronic acid to chondroitin sulfate (21).

The indurated character of the dermal syphilomas—with rubbery consistency suggests that they contain chondroitin-like tissue in relatively large amounts, and limited chemical analyses in this laboratory support this view. Because of the known presence of substantial amounts of hyaluronic acid in early dermal syphilomas of rabbits, the subsequent development of cartilaginous-like tissue, and the rapid changes in either direction when cortisone is given or withdrawn, the hypothesis is advanced that this indurated tissue is formed by the conversion of the treponemal hyaluronic acid to a sulfated molecule of the nature of chondroitin sulfate.

Layton (22), utilizing radioactive tracer techniques, has shown that sulfate in abnormal amounts is fixed in injured muscle tissue and in granulation tissue in a number of animal species. The same investigator (23) has also obtained evidence that sulfate fixation in injured tissue is inhibited by cortisone. By analogy it might be further postulated that in cortisone-treated rabbits sulfating of hyaluronic acid is interfered with, either indirectly through removal of the cellular elements or by some more direct inhibition of the enzyme system concerned, thus permitting accumulation of the nonsulfated mucopolysaccharide.[5] Such a hypothesis appears to be consistent with the observed sequence of events, although it admittedly rests on meagre experimental evidence.

A third notable feature of cortisone effect on dermal syphilomas is the rebound phenomenon observed upon the withdrawal of cortisone. This usually occurs within forty-eight hours after the last dose is given, but in exceptional instances it may be delayed a number of days. Considering the fact that the lesions contain an excessive number of treponemes as a result of cortisone therapy, it is not surprising that the discontinuance of cortisone is followed by an unusually severe form of disease as manifested by extensive local and generalized lesions. After long-continued cortisone therapy no rebound is observed in about half

---

[5] Interesting studies on this general subject have also been recently reported by H. Boström, and B. Månsson. On the enxymatic exchange of the sulfate group of chondroitinsulfuric acid in slices of cartilage, *J. Biol. Chem.*, 1952, 196, 483.

the animals, which may be accounted for by the development of protective antibody.

The evidence suggests, therefore, that the most striking effect of cortisone therapy on syphilomas in rabbits is less dependent upon inhibition of antibody formation than upon a direct effect on the tissues at the point of contact between parasite and host and that a prominent feature of this effect is alteration in the ratio of hyaluronic acid and chondroitin-sulfate.

Summary.—The administration of cortisone to rabbits with dermal syphilomas profoundly alters the character of the lesions and to a lesser extent the subsequent course of the disease. In contrast to the usual reddish, indurated, and often stony hard lesions, those in cortisone-treated animals are pale, soft, and filled with a tenacious mucoid material identified as hyaluronic acid. *T. pallidum* occurs in such lesions in excessive numbers.

Upon withdrawal of cortisone there is a rebound phenomenon characterized by a return of the lesions to their pre treatment characteristics, except that they usually become much larger than in animals which have received no cortisone. Generalized syphilitic lesions occur in a much higher proportion of cortisone-treated animals than in untreated rabbits.

Partly on evidence adduced in these experiments, the hypothesis is advanced that the most striking effect of cortisone therapy on the lesions in this experimental infection is less dependent upon inhibition of antibody formation than upon a direct effect on the tissues at the point of contact between the parasite and the host, so that the removal of treponemal hyaluronic acid is inhibited and a prominent feature of this effect is an alteration of the ratio of hyaluronic acid and chondroitin-sulfate.

REFERENCES

1. Turner, T. B., and D. H. Hollander, Cortisone in experimental syphilis (A preliminary note), *Bull. Johns Hopkins Hosp.*, 1950, 87:5.
2. Magnuson, H. J., H. Eagle, and R. Fleischman, The minimal infectious inoculum of spirochaeta pallida (Nichols strain), and a consideration of its rate of multiplication in vivo, *Am. J. Syph., Gon. & V. D.*, 1948, 32:1.
3. Cumberland, M. C., and T. B. Turner, The rate of multiplication of *T. pallidum* in normal and immune rabbits, *Am. J. Syph., Gon. & V. D.*, 1949, 33:201.

4. Hollander, D. H., T. B. Turner, and E. E. Nell, The effect of long continued subcurative doses of penicillin during the incubation period of experimental syphilis, Bull. Johns Hopkins Hosp., 1952, 90:105.
5. Scott, V., and G. Dammin, Hyaluronidase and experimental syphilis; III: Metachromasia in syphilitic orchitis and its relationship to hyaluronic acid, Am. J. Syph., Gon. & V. D., 1950, 34:501.
6. Turner, T. B., M. C. Cumberland, and H.-Y Li, Comparative effectiveness of penicillins G, F, K, and X in experimental syphilis as determined by a short in vivo method, Am. J. Syph., Gon. & V. D., 1947, 31:476.
7. Turner, T. B., and R. A. Nelson, Jr., The relationship of treponemal immobilizing antibody to immunity in syphilis, Trans. Assoc. Amer. Phys., 1950, 63:112.
8. Chesney, A. M., and G. F. Schipper, The effect of the method of inoculation upon the course of experimental syphilis in the rabbit, Am. J. Syph., Gonor. & V. D., 1950, 34:18.
9. DeLamater, E. D., V. Saurino, and F. Urbach, Studies on the immunology of spirochetosis; I: Effect of cortisone on experimental spirochetosis, Am. J. Syph., Gon. & V. D., 1952, 36:127.
10. Pearce, R. H., and E. M. Watson, The mucopolysaccharides of human skin, Canad. J. Res. (Section E), 1949, 27:43.
11. Einbinder, J., and M. Schubert, Separation of chondroitin sulfate from cartilage, J. Biol. Chem., 1950, 185:725.
12. Jeanloz, R. W., and E. Forchielli, Studies on hyaluronic acid and related substances; I: Preparation of hyaluronic acid and derivatives from human umbilical cord, J. Biol. Chem., 1950, 186:495.
13. Stacey, M., The chemistry of mucopolysaccharides and mucoproteins, Advances in Carbohydrate Chemistry, 1946, 2:161.
14. White, A., Effects of adrenal steroids on blood cells and on certain aspects of protein metabolism, in Symposium on Steroid Hormones, 1950, pp. 195–211.
15. Ragan, C., and others, Effect of cortisone on production of granulation tissue in the rabbit, Proc. Soc. Exp. Biol. & Med., 1949, 72:718.
16. Adlersberg, D., L. E. Schaeffer, and R. Dritch, Adrenal cortex and lipid metabolism; effects of cortisone and adrenocorticotropin (ACTH) on serum lipids in man, Proc. Soc. Exp. Biol. & Med., 1950, 74:877.
17. Rich, A. R., T. H. Cochran, and D. C. McGoon, Marked lipemia resulting from the administration of cortisone, Bull. Johns Hopkins Hosp., 1951, 88:101.
18. Molomut, N., D. M. Spain, and A. Haber, The effects of cortisone on the spleen in mice, Proc. Soc. Exp. Biol. & Med., 1950, 73:416.
19. McLeod, C. M., The mode of action of mucin in experimental meningococcus infection; II: The effect of the defense mechanism of the mouse, Am. J. Hyg., 1941, 34:B51.
20. Duran-Reynals, F., Introduction: The ground substance of the mesenchyme and hyaluronidase, Ann. N.Y. Acad. Sci., 1950, 52:943.

21. Watson, E. M., and R. H. Pearce, The cutaneous mucopolysaccharides in localized (pretibial) myxedema, *Ann. N.Y. Acad. Sci.*, 1950, 52:1004.
22. Layton, L. L., In vitro sulfate fixation by granulation tissue and injured muscle tissue from healing wounds, *Proc. Soc. Exp. Biol. & Med.* 1950, 73:570.
23. Layton, L. L., Effect of cortisone upon chondroitin sulfate synthesis by animal tissues, *Proc. Soc. Exp. Biol. & Med.*, 1951, 76:596.

Chapter 10

THE EFFECT OF CORTISONE IN ACTIVATING LATENT TRYPANOSOMIASIS IN RHESUS MONKEYS [1]

By Abner Wolf, Elvin A. Kabat, Ada E. Bezer, and James R. C. Fonseca, *The Departments of Pathology, Neurology, and Microbiology, College of Physicians and Surgeons, Columbia University, and the Neurological Institute, Presbyterian Hospital, New York*

During the course of experiments on the effect of cortisone on acute disseminated encephalomyelitis produced experimentally in rhesus monkeys by the injection of homologous brain tissue emulsified with the Freund adjuvants (1), it was noted that the cortisone activated a spontaneous latent infection by trypanosomes. The seventy-nine Macaccus rhesus monkeys used were Indian in origin and were obtained from a New York dealer during the winter of 1950. In examining blood specimens from the monkeys to determine their eosinophile content, motile flagellates were noted in the blood of six of the eight animals investigated. Two were control animals which had received no cortisone, and four were cortisone treated. A study of the organism in blood smears showed it to be a trypanosome, roughly 19–20 micra. in length, with a large posterior kinetoplast, very finely granular, lightly basophilic cytoplasm, a good-sized flagellum and a narrow undulating membrane (Fig. 1). In wet preparations the trypanosomes were strikingly active and motile.

The administration of cortisone was begun a week prior to the injection of the brain emulsions with adjuvants. Each monkey, cortisone-treated or control, had a series of three inoculations of 1 ml. per dose of monkey brain, aquaphor, paraffin oil, and heat-killed tubercle bacilli given at weekly intervals. The emulsion of monkey brain with the Freund adjuvants was prepared as formerly reported (2). Fifty-nine monkeys received cortisone subcutaneously, while twenty animals re-

---

[1] Aided by a grant (MH-257) from the National Institute of Mental Health of the National Institutes of Health, Public Health Service, and by the William J. Matheson Commission; an abstract of this work appeared in *Federation Proceedings*, 1951, 10, 375.

ceived none. Cortisone was given daily to six animals, and six times weekly to fifty-three others while the brain injections were under way and for eight weeks thereafter, a total of eleven weeks of cortisone administration. In some groups of animals cortisone was discontinued

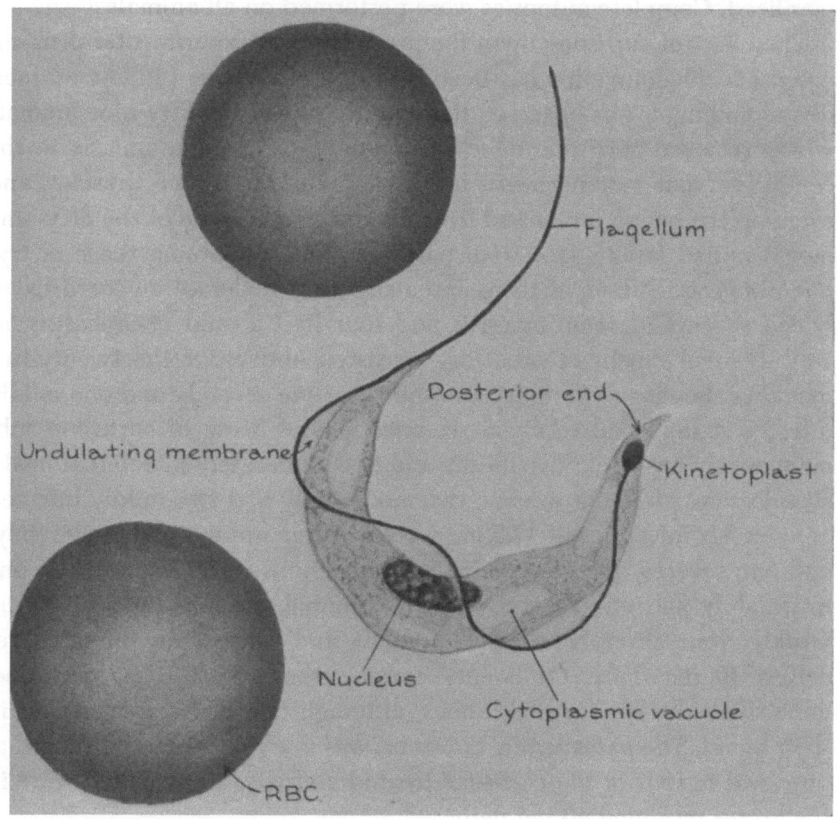

FIGURE 1. TRYPANOSOME SEEN IN SMEAR OF BLOOD OF CORTISONE-TREATED RHESUS MONKEY
Note size of flagellate in relation to red blood cells and terminal position and large size of blepharoplast; probably T. cruzi.

after administration for three to six weeks. Animals were observed daily for signs of illness. Those which showed such grave signs of encephalomyelitis that they seemed unlikely to survive another day were sacrificed. Ataxia, visual loss, and pyramidal tract signs were the most common signs. Comparison with later autopsy findings revealed that they probably resulted from the experimentally produced disseminated encephalomyelitis, and not from the protozoan infection. Weakness and loss of weight in the protozoan-infected animals were in part caused by the cortisone. At the termination of the experiment, eight weeks after the last injection of brain emulsion, all the remaining monkeys were sacrificed. Complete autopsies were performed on all animals.

The effect of cortisone upon the production of experimental disseminated encephalomyelitis has been reported elsewhere (1). As an incidental finding, it was observed that twenty-two of the fifty-nine animals which received cortisone developed lesions of trypanosomiasis in the central nervous system, heart, fat, bone marrow, striated muscles, and rarely in the lymph nodes and liver. In addition, sixteen of the fifty-nine monkeys had lesions free from parasites, but resembling those of trypanosomiasis. Fifteen of them had a slight or moderate myocarditis, of which seven had some myositis and four had a mild encephalitis, as well as involvement of other organs listed above. Of the twenty-two monkeys showing definite trypanosomiasis, one severely and one mildly infected animal had received six injections of 5 mg of cortisone subcutaneously per week; two mildly and two moderately infected animals, six injections of 10 mg weekly; two moderately and two mildly infected animals, six injections of 17.5 mg weekly; three mildly, one moderately, and one severely infected animal, six injections of 20 mg weekly; one moderately and one severely infected animal, six injections of 30 mg weekly; four severely infected animals and one mildly infected received 40 mg daily. Of twenty animals that received no cortisone, none showed trypanosomal lesions, although two had trypanosomes in their blood. The parasitemia, however, was much less marked than that observed in four of the cortisone-treated animals, all of which were in the group receiving 40 mg daily.

Pathological Findings

Nervous System.—Focal inflammatory lesions were scattered throughout the brain and spinal cord. They were encountered most often in the cerebral cortex, but were also seen in the cerebral white matter, basal ganglia, hypothalamus, cerebellum, brain stem, and spinal cord, being present in both gray and white matter at all levels of the neuraxis. The chief feature of the process was a miliary granuloma (Fig. 2). This was composed of a cluster of large, rounded, ovoid, polygonal, or fusiform cells, with abundant cytoplasm and eccentric or central oval nuclei, poor in chromatin and often having a prominent nucleolus (Fig. 3). Leishmaniform organisms were present in the cytoplasm of these cells (Fig. 3), varying from a few to a large number which completely filled the cell and displaced its nucleus toward the cell margin. These organisms lay in cytoplasmic vacuoles and averaged about 2 micra in length. They were ovoid or spherical in shape and had an oval or spherical

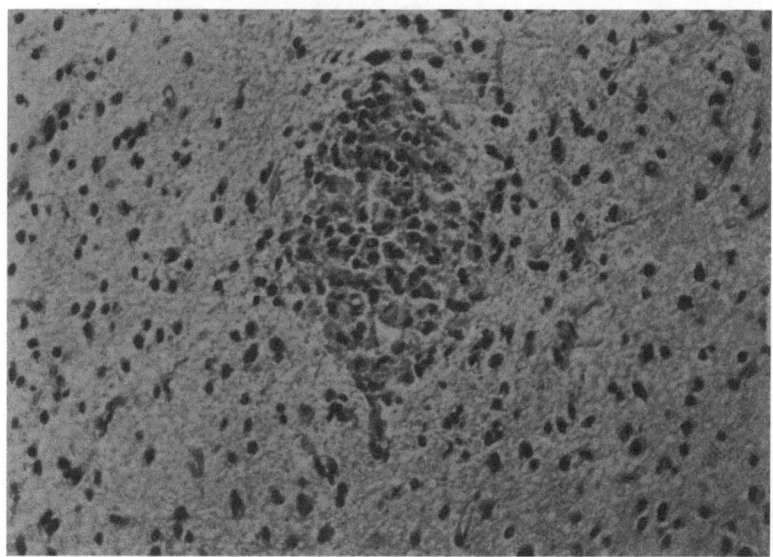

FIGURE 2. MILIARY GRANULOMA IN CORTEX OF FRONTAL LOBE OF CEREBRUM OF RHESUS MONKEY SUFFERING FROM TRYPANOSOMIASIS
Hematoxylin eosin stain ×100.

nucleus and a rod-like transverse blepharoplast (Fig. 4). The miliary granulomas usually exhibited an intimate relationship to a small blood vessel, commonly a capillary, which showed hypertrophy and cytoplasmic basophilia of its endothelial lining cells. Nerve cells and fibers were included in the outer portions of the granulomas and usually were remarkably well preserved. The largest of the granulomas, resulting from a coalescence of smaller ones, compressed the surrounding neural tissue to a mild degree, and this was associated with some distortion, edema of the parenchyma, and a mild astrocytosis. Perivascular lymphocytes were encountered in small numbers about the granulomas with an occasional plasma cell and large mononuclear cell. When the granuloma was near the surface, the overlying leptomeninges showed a similar, mild, strictly limited infiltration. Even the largest granulomas were a mm or less in diameter, and some of them had undergone central necrosis (Fig. 5) associated with some polymorphonuclear infiltration.

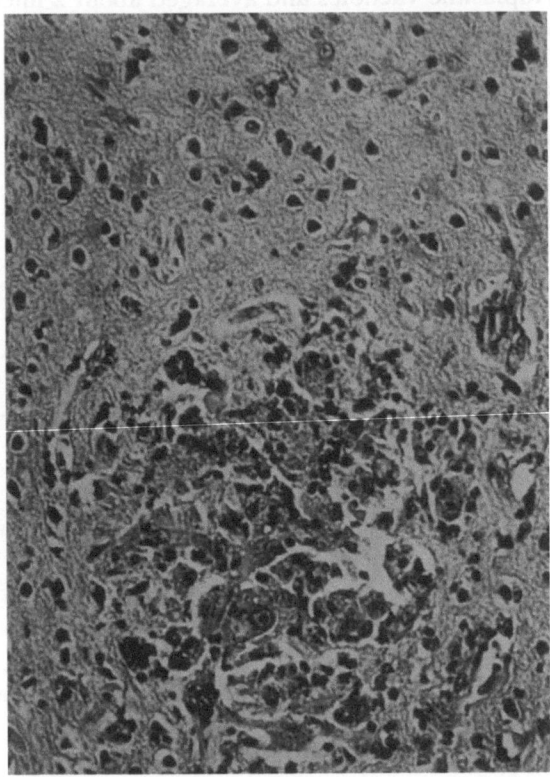

FIGURE 3. MILIARY GRANULOMA IN CORTEX OF OCCIPITAL LOBE OF CEREBRUM OF RHESUS MONKEY WITH TRYPANOSOMIASIS
Marked parasitization of epithelioid cells by leishmaniform stage of trypanosome; hematoxylin eosin stain ×100.

In these granulomatous lesions leishmaniform organisms were seen extracellularly, and perivascular infiltration was somewhat more intense. In only one monkey, one which had received 40 mg of cortisone daily and had a severe trypanasomal encephalomyelitis, was another type of lesion found. In this animal a portion of the cortex of one occipital lobe showed advanced degeneration extending down into the subcortical white matter. The cortex was narrowed and its architecture was vir-

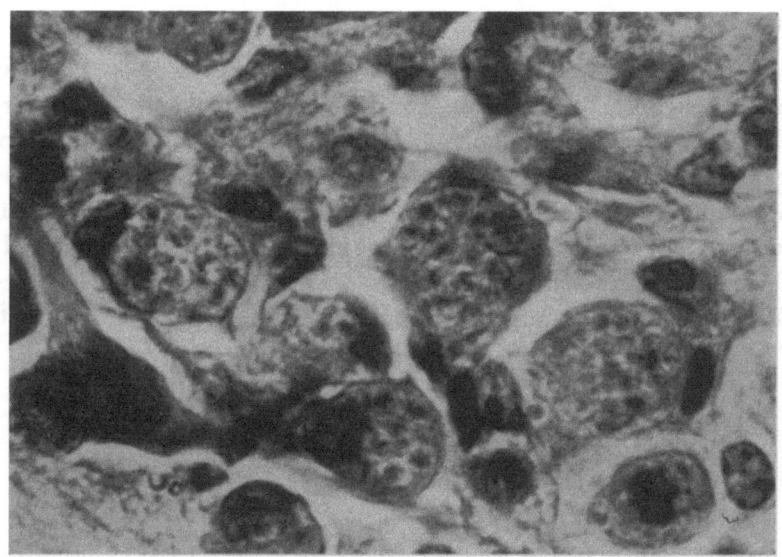

FIGURE 4. LEISHMANIFORM STAGE OF TRYPANOSOME IN LARGE MONO-
NUCLEAR ELEMENTS IN FOCAL LESION OF CEREBRAL CORTEX OF
RHESUS MONKEY WITH TRYPANOSOMIASIS
Hematoxylin eosin stain ×1000.

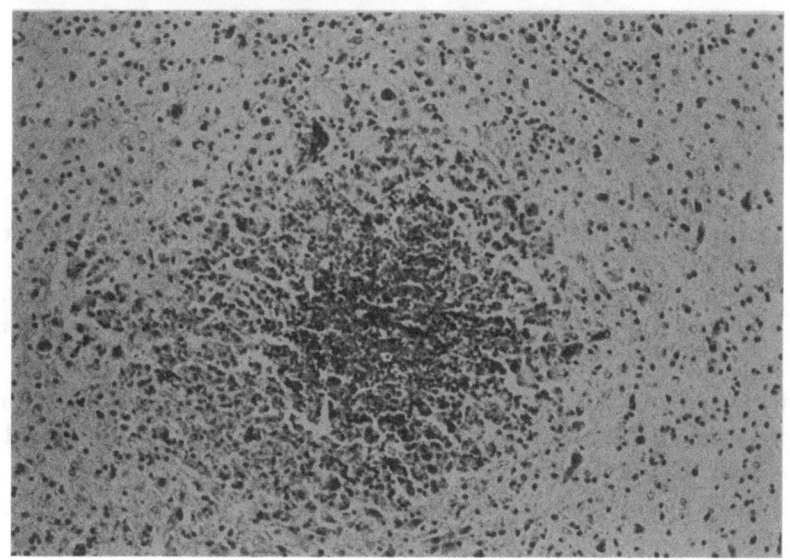

FIGURE 5. LARGE GRANULOMA IN CORTEX OF FRONTAL LOBE OF
CEREBRUM OF RHESUS MONKEY WITH TRYPANOSOMIASIS, SHOW-
ING EXTENSIVE CENTRAL NECROSIS
Hematoxylin eosin stain ×50.

tually obliterated because of extensive loss of nerve cells. There was some microgliosis, in the form of rod-cell formation, and intense large-cell astrocytosis. Large mononuclear cells, loaded with leishmaniform organisms, were present in perivascular spaces, and there was a moderate capillary endothelial hyperplasia. In one area total disorganization, with cyst formation and marginal fibrillary astrocytosis, marked by reduced cellularity and piloid forms, was the site of many coalescent miliary granulomas containing numerous organisms (Fig. 6). Astro-

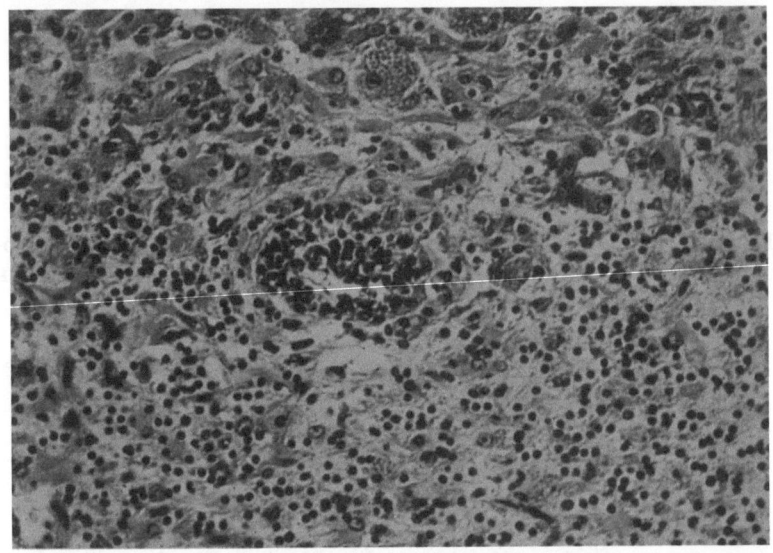

FIGURE 6. SEVERE TRYPANOSOMAL LESION IN CEREBRAL CORTEX OF RHESUS MONKEY
Total destruction of neural elements, coalescence of granulomas, lymphocytosis, and numerous intracellular leishmaniform organisms; hematoxylin eosin stain ×100.

cytes were found richly garlanding the granulomas. Perivascular and leptomeningeal infiltration, as described above, was more marked in this area. In another heavily infected animal, one which had also received 40 mg of cortisone daily, leishmaniform organisms were found in the cytoplasm of arachnoid cells and dural histiocytes in one optic nerve sheath. Lymphocytes were present in the leptomeningeal portion of the sheath. In another animal a centrally necrotic granuloma was seen in a posterior root at a lumbar level.

A number of nerves of the brachial plexus in one of the most severely infected animals, an animal which had received 40 mg of cortisone daily, showed focal lesions in the perineurium and endoneurium. Large mononuclear cells, parasitized by leishmaniform organisms, were seen perivascularly. These occurred singly or in clusters, but were discrete, and did not form compact granulomas, as in the central nervous system. They were associated with moderate numbers of lymphocytes, proliferating capillaries and a multiplication of local sheath cells. No focal degeneration of axones or myelin sheaths was observed. Leishmaniform organisms, with a lesser inflammatory reaction, were seen in the perineurium and endoneurium of the sciatic nerves and brachial plexuses of a number of other animals.

Heart.—There was a focal or diffuse interstitial myocarditis most marked in the ventricles (Fig. 7). An interstitial infiltration by lymphocytes and occasional plasma cells was accompanied by capillary proliferation and multiplication of histiocytes. Dense clusters of leishmaniform organisms were seen in muscle fibers in these areas (Fig. 8) and beyond them. The muscle fibers were often pressed widely apart by

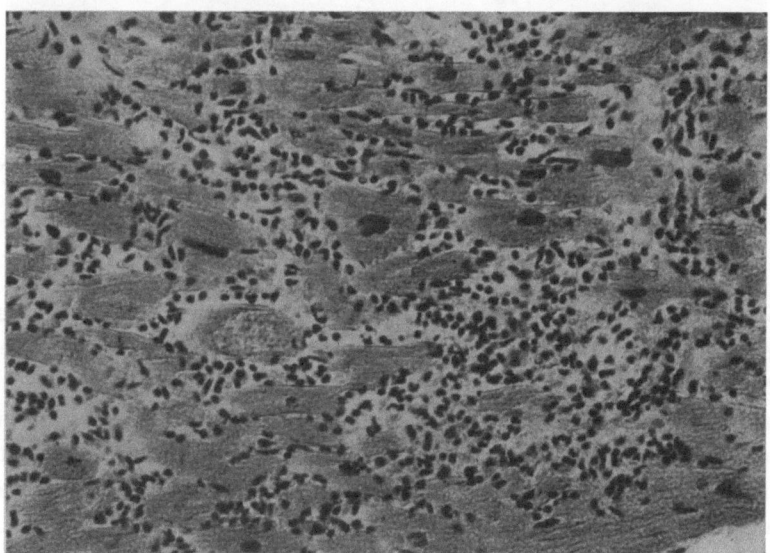

FIGURE 7. INTERSTITIAL TRYPANOSOMAL MYOCARDITIS IN RHESUS MONKEY
Note infestation of muscle fibers by leishmaniform organisms and the interstitial infiltration by lymphocytes; hematoxylin eosin stain ×100.

the interstitial inflammation. Granular degeneration of myocardial fibers was seen only in the most severe lesions. Wherever the lesions were superficial there was focal extension of the inflammation into the pericardium. In one instance focal subendocardial necrosis of connective tissue, with localized polymorphonuclear infiltration, was observed.

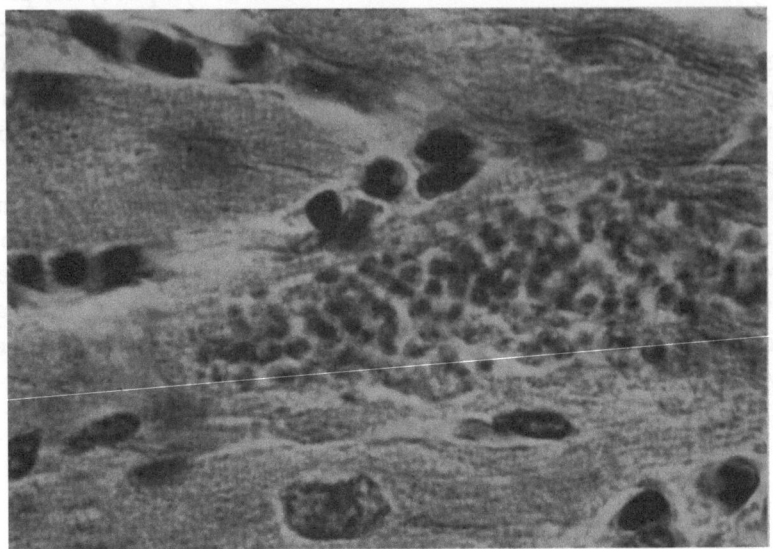

FIGURE 8. DENSE CLUSTER OF LEISHMANIFORM ORGANISMS IN MUSCLE FIBER; TRYPANOSOMAL MYOCARDITIS IN RHESUS MONKEY
Hematoxylin eosin stain ×1000.

Striated muscle.—Interstitial inflammation like that seen in the heart was present here, as well (Fig. 9). Many of the closely packed mononuclear cells, which were considered to be proliferating histiocytes, resembled epithelioid elements. Many muscle fibers were filled with leishmaniform organisms (Fig. 9). Focal hyaline and granular degeneration of muscle fibers was accompanied by swelling and loss of striation. Multiplication of muscle and sarcolemma nuclei was observed, and occasional multinucleated basophilic fibers gave evidence of attempts at regeneration.

Fat.—Subcutaneous and peritoneal fat contained focal areas of infiltration by lymphocytes and large mononuclear elements (Fig. 10) parasitized by leishmaniform organisms (Fig. 11) and had the same

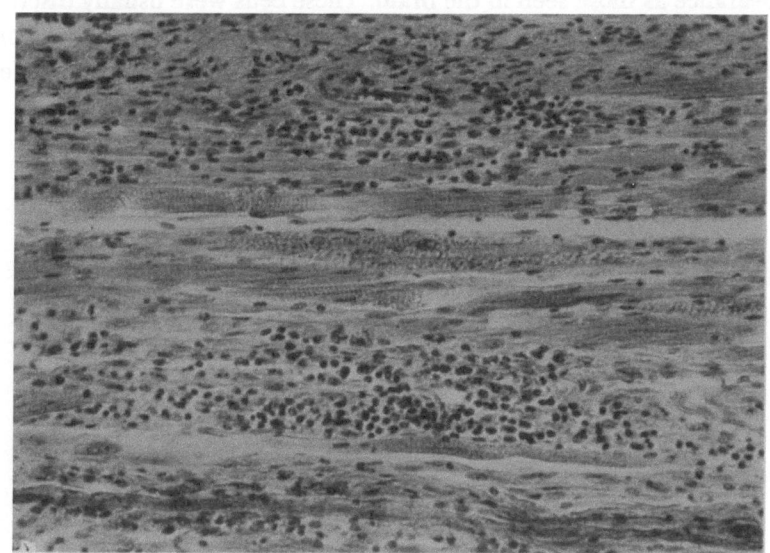

FIGURE 9. TRYPANOSOMAL MYOSITIS IN RHESUS MONKEY
Hematoxylin eosin stain ×100.

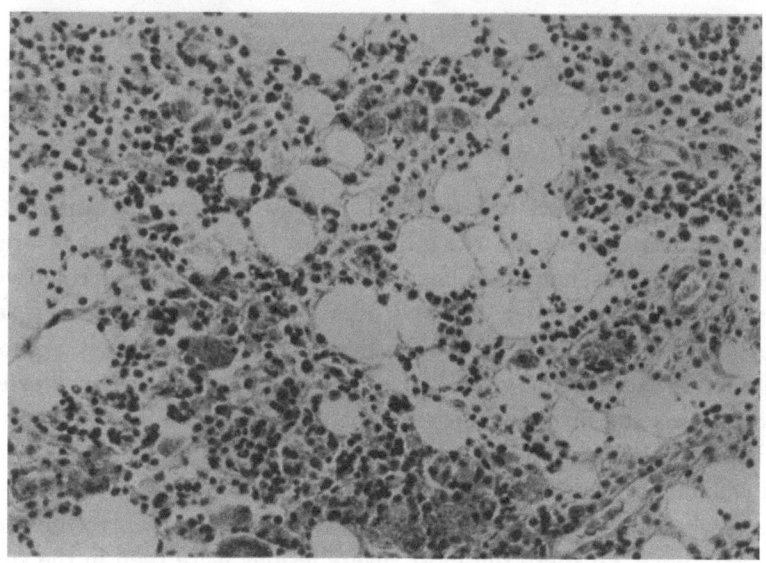

FIGURE 10. FOCAL TRYPANOSOMAL LESIONS IN SUBCUTANEOUS FAT IN RHESUS MONKEY
Hematoxylin eosin stain ×100.

appearance as those seen in the brain. These cells were usually discrete, but sometimes occurred in denser clusters, in which they were polygonal, rounded, or fusiform. Occasionally a few polymorphonuclear leucocytes were seen in foci of fat necrosis.

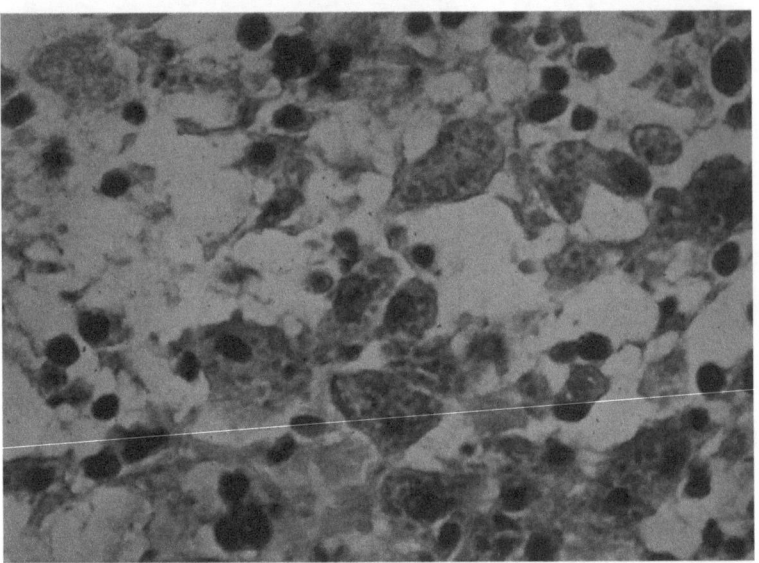

FIGURE 11. LARGE MONONUCLEAR ELEMENTS PARASITIZED BY LEISHMANIFORM ORGANISMS IN TRYPANOSOMAL LESION IN SUBCUTANEOUS FAT OF RHESUS MONKEY
Hematoxylin eosin stain ×400.

Bone marrow.—Foci of large mononuclear elements parasitized by leishmaniform organisms resembled those seen in the fat. Normal myeloid elements had disappeared, and the mononuclear cells were accompanied by lymphocytes and occasional polymorphonuclear leucocytes. The parasitized mononuclear cells did not lie closely approximated as in the cerebral granulomas, but lay more discretely in clusters. Focal necroses of marrow were encountered, with few, if any, organisms and some polymorphonuclear leucocytes.

Involvement of the intestine, liver, and lymph nodes was rare and was marked by chronic focal inflammatory lesions similar to those described above. Of these the most severe lesions were seen in the small intestine of one animal in which all layers were involved, but the submucosa and mucosa were chiefly affected.

LATENT TRYPANOSOMIASIS

Discussion.—In view of the finding of a trypanosome in the blood of some of the animals in this experimental group, it was clear that the microorganisms observed in their tissues were the leishmaniform stage of the flagellate. Unfortunately, by the time the pathological observations were made, the trypanosome was no longer available for studies as to its pathogenicity by inoculation into other species.

The occurrence of spontaneous trypanosomiasis in monkeys was first noted in 1908 independently by Gonder and Von Berenberg-Gossler (3) in South America and by Brumpt (4) in 1909 in Belgium. Gonder and Von Berenberg-Gossler observed these flagellates in Brachyurus calvus monkeys in the Amazon district and named them Trypanosoma prowazeki. Later, Laveran and Mesnil (5) and Malamos (6) expressed the opinion that the illustrations of the organisms in this report strongly suggested Trypanosoma cruzi. Brumpt found his trypanosomes in a young Macaccus cynomolgous monkey from the zoological garden of Antwerp and named it Trypanosoma vickersae. It was very similar to Trypanosoma cruzi. It was easily transmissible and was passaged to six cynomolgous, one Maccus sinicus, and one Macaccus rhesus monkey, two guinea pigs and three young rabbits, with no occurrence of symptoms. Brumpt later concluded that it was pathogenic in some respects and was responsible for the death of a few of his monkeys. In 1911 Terry (7) found actively motile trypanosomes in the blood of twenty-eight Macaccus rhesus monkeys at the Rockefeller Institute, New York City, and was able to transmit them to one Macaccus rhesus monkey, six mice, two rats and a guinea pig. He found the organism to be only mildly pathogenic, and tentatively named it Trypanosoma rhesi. Laveran and Mesnil (5) suggested that this organism was the same as that described by Brumpt (4). In 1918 Leger and Porry (8) found a trypanosome in an Ateles pendadactylus monkey in French Guinea which they named Trypanosoma lesourdi; they were unable to transmit it to monkeys or to guinea pigs. In 1935 Malamos (6) observed trypanosomes identified as Schizotrypanum cruzi in four Javanese cynomolgous monkeys recently received in Hamburg. The infection was transmitted to monkeys, mice, and rats; Triatoma infestans could be infected by blood sucking. In 1946 Fulton and Harrison (9) reported on a batch of Macaccus rhesus monkeys which they had received from India for a study of malaria. Following a series of blood inoculations from one to another of the group, six animals were found to harbor trypanosomes in their blood, described as indistinguishable from a strain of Trypansoma cruzi maintained in the laboratory. Some sickened and died, two very suddenly. Lesions were encountered in the liver, spleen, heart, pericardium, and bone marrow. Fulton and Harrison also cited a personal communication from MacCallum (10) stating that he had found Trypanosoma cruzi in the blood of some Macaccus rhesus monkeys which had been in his laboratory for some time. In the recent edition of Brumpt's textbook of parasitology (11) he stated the opinion that the typanosome described by him in the Javanese monkey in 1909, that by Terry in Indian monkeys in 1911, and that in Dutch East Indian monkeys by Malamos in 1935 were all examples of the Trypanosoma cruzi of Chagas. Fulton and Harrison and MacCallum also considered their organisms to be T. cruzi. It is highly probable, although certainly not proved, that the trypanosome in our monkeys, like those in these other Indian monkeys is also T. cruzi. This probability is increased by the predominance of lesions in the central nervous system and heart. The striking tendency to granuloma formation in the central nervous system, with clusters of large epithelioid cells containing the leishmaniform stage of the organism, is very similar to that seen in human Chagas disease. The granulomas are relatively free of lymphocytes, show no giant cells, and only rarely exhibit necrosis. Focal necrotizing lesions are fewer. In the heart, the lively interstitial myocarditis, marked by the predominance of round cells and the leishmaniform organisms in the muscle fibers, is the essential lesion. A similar, less-marked involvement of striated muscle is present. The bone marrow is strikingly affected and exhibits both necrotizing and granulomatous lesions, as does the fat, but to a lesser degree.

In general it was found that the higher the dose of cortisone the more severe the trypanosomal infection, particularly the encephalomyelitis and myocarditis. Conversely, the experimental disseminated encephalomyelitis produced by the inoculation of an emulsion of brain tissue and Freund adjuvants was eliminated by the higher doses of cortisone and occurred sporadically and less markedly with succeeding smaller doses. The presence of the experimental encephalomyelitis did not appear to favor the development of trypanosomiasis or seem to affect its degree. In view of the fact that twenty-two of the monkeys which received cortisone showed trypanosomal lesions and organisms and another sixteen had similar lesions without the organisms, out of a total of fifty-nine receiving this medication, and that twenty other monkeys treated in exactly the same way, but having no cortisone administered, were free of trypanosomal lesions, except for latent blood infection in two, one may conclude that the cortisone activated a latent trypanosomiasis in these animals.

The histological character of the lesions produced by the trypanosomes did not appear to be modified by the cortisone as determined by a cross comparison with available material of simian trypanosomiasis. There were changes in a number of organs due to the cortisone administration, however. The adrenal glands showed narrowing of their cortices, with a depletion of lipids. Their spleens exhibited quiescent Malpighian corpuscles and a red pulp poor in cellular elements. The lymph nodes were relatively inactive, and the thymus glands scanty in volume and inactive. This was in contrast to the findings in the monkeys having received no cortisone, which for the most part developed experimental disseminated encephalomyelitis and showed no lesions of trypanosomiasis. These had broad adrenal cortices, which appeared active and contained an abundance of lipid. Their spleens had Malpighian corpuscles with active germinal centers and a cellular red pulp. The lymph nodes exhibited active germinal follicles and many mononuclear cells in their medulla. Often the thymus was large and active or of moderate size.

The stimulation of a more vigorous trypanosomiasis in monkeys harboring an inapparent parasitization of this type by the administration of cortisone extends the repeated observation of the enhancing effect of this substance on spontaneous and experimentally induced infections. Many of these are discussed in detail in the other papers of this symposium (12–40). The mechanism by which these effects on infections are produced have not yet been definitely determined. The well-known metabolic influence of cortisone and its effects on lymphoid tissue, especially the recently established role in wound healing (41–46), inflammation, capillary permeability, and phagocytosis (47–51), antibody formation (52), and various allergic reactions (53–54) provide good leads for further study. Many of them have been evaluated in detail in other contributions to this symposium.

Summary.—Fifty-nine Macaccus rhesus monkeys were given cortisone in order to observe its effect upon the development of acute disseminated encephalomyelitis produced by the inoculation of homologous brain tissue emulsified with the Freund adjuvants, and twenty served as control animals. Twenty-two of the fifty-nine of the cortisone-treated monkeys developed lesions of trypanosomiasis (probably caused by T. cruzi) in the central nervous system, heart, fat, bone marrow, striated muscle, and rarely in the lymph nodes and liver. In addition, sixteen of the fifty-nine monkeys had lesions free of parasites, but resembling those of trypanosomiasis. The twenty control animals which did not receive cortisone and most of which developed experimental acute disseminated encephalomyelitis, were all free of trypanosomal lesions, although two had a parasitemia. These findings provide additional evidence that cortisone enhances the infection caused by a variety of infectious agents.

REFERENCES

1. Kabat, E. A., A. Wolf, and A. E. Bezer, Studies on acute disseminated encephalomyelitis produced experimentally in rhesus monkeys; VII: The effect of cortisone, *J. Immunol.*, 1952, 68:265.
2. —— Rapid production of acute disseminated encephalomyelitis in rhesus monkeys by injection of heterologous and homologous brain tissue with adjuvants, *J. Exp. Med.*, 1947, 85:117.
3. Gonder, R., and H. von Berenberg-Gossler, Untersuchungen ueber Malariaplasmodien der Affen, *Malaria*, 1908–9, 1:47.
4. Brumpt, E., Sur un nouveau trypanosome non pathogène du singe, *Bull. de la Soc. de path. exot.*, 1909, 2:267.
5. Laveran, A., and F. Mesnil, Trypanosomes et trypanosomiasis. 2d ed. Masson et Cie, Paris, 1912.
6. Malamos, B., Ueber Vorkommen von Schizotrypanum cruzi bei Affen in Niederländisch Indien, *Arch. F. Schiffs u. Tropen. Hyg.*, 1935, 39:156.
7. Terry, B. T., Trypanosomiasis in monkeys (Macaccus rhesus) in captivity, *Proc. Soc. Exp. Biol. & Med.*, 1911, 9:17.
8. Leger, M., and E. Porry, Trypanosomes nouveaux de deux singes de la Guyanne francaise, *Compt. rend. hebdom. Soc. de Biol.*, 1918, 81:180.
9. Fulton, J. D., and C. V. Harrison, An outbreak of Trypanosoma cruzi infection in Indian monkeys, *Tr. Roy. Soc. Trop. Med. & Hyg.*, 1946, 39:513.
10. MacCallum, F. O., Personal communication to Fulton and Harrison (9).
11. Brumpt, E., Précis de parastologie; collection de précis medicaux. 6th ed. Masson et Cie, Paris, 1949.
12. Shwartzman, G., Enhancing effect of cortisone upon poliomyelitis infection (strain MEF_1) in hamsters and mice, *Proc. Soc. Exp. Biol. & Med.*, 1950, 85:835.
13. Kilbourne, E. D., and F. L. Horsfall, Increased virus in eggs injected with cortisone, *Proc. Soc. Exp. Biol. & Med.*, 1951, 76:116.

14. —— Lethal infection with Coxsackie virus of adult mice given cortisone, *Proc. Soc. Exp. Biol. & Med.*, 1951, 77:135.
15. Southam, C. M., and V. I. Babcock, Effect of cortisone, related hormones, and adrenalectomy on susceptibility of mice to virus infections, *Proc. Soc. Exp. Biol. & Med.*, 1951, 78:105.
16. Vollmer, E. P., and H. S. Hurlbut, Ineffectiveness of cortisone therapy in mice infected with Japanese B encephalitis and the adverse effect of high doses, *J. Inf. Dis.*, 1951, 89:103.
17. Loosli, C. G., R. B. Hull, B. S. Berlin, and E. R. Alexander, The influence of ACTH on the course of experimental influenza type A virus infection, *J. Lab. & Clin. Med.*, 1951, 37:464.
18. Kalter, S. S., H. I. Smolin, J. M. McElhaney, and J. Tepperman, Endocrines and their relation to influenza virus infection, *J. Exp. Med.*, 1951, 93:529.
19. Kass, E. H., S. H. Ingbar, M. M. Lundgren, and M. Finland, The effect of ACTH and cortisone on pneumococcal and influenza viral infections in the white mouse, *J. Lab. & Clin. Med.*, 1951, 37:780.
20. Jackson, E. B., and J. E. Smadel, Cortisone and ACTH on toxins of rickettsiae and salmonella typhosa, *Proc. Soc. Amer. Bact.*, 1950, p. 92.
21. Antopol, W., Anatomic changes produced in mice treated with excessive doses of cortisone, *Proc. Soc. Exp. Biol. & Med.*, 1950, 73:262.
22. Antopol, W., S. Glaubach, and H. Quittner, Experimental observations with massive doses of cortisone, *Rheumatism*, 1951, 8:1.
23. Selye, H., The influence of STH, ACTH and cortisone upon resistance to infection, *Canad. Med. J.*, 1951, 64:489.
24. Le Maistre, C., and R. Tompsett, The emergence of pseudotuberculosis in rats given cortisone, *J. Exp. Med.*, 1952, 95:393.
25. Spain, D. M. and N. Molomut, Effects of cortisone on the development of tuberculous lesions in guinea pigs and on their modification by streptomycin therapy. *Am. Rev. Tuberc.*, 1950, 62:337.
26. Michaelis, M., M. M. Cummings, and W. L. Bloom, Course of experimental tuberculosis in the albino rat as influenced by cortisone, *Proc. Soc. Exp. Biol. & Med.*, 1950, 75:613.
27. Hart, P. d'Arcy, and R. J. W. Rees, Enhancing effect of cortisone on tuberculosis in the mouse, *Lancet*, 1950, 2:391.
28. Lurie, M. B., P. Zappasodi, and A. M. Dannenberg, Constitutional factors in resistance to infection: the effect of cortisone on the pathogenesis of tuberculosis, *Science*, 1951, 113:234.
29. Bloch, R. G., K. Vennesland, and C. Gurney, The effect of cortisone on tuberculosis in the guinea pig, *J. Lab. & Clin. Med.*, 1951, 38:133.
30. Solotorovsky, M., F. J. Gregory, and H. C. Stoerk, Loss of protection by vaccination following cortisone treatment in mice with experimentally induced tuberculosis, *Proc. Soc. Exp. Biol. & Med.*, 1951, 76:286.
31. Mogabgab, W. J., and L. Thomas, The effects of cortisone on experi-

mental infection with group A streptococci in rabbits, *J. Lab. & Clin. Med.*, 1950, 36:968.
32. Kligman, A. M., D. Baldridge, G. Rebell, and D. M. Pillsbury, The effect of cortisone on the pathologic responses of guinea pigs infected cutaneously with fungi, viruses and bacteria, *J. Lab. & Clin. Med.*, 1951, 37:615.
33. Turner, T. B., and D. H. Hollander, Cortisone in experimental syphilis; a preliminary note, *Bull. Johns Hopkins Hosp.*, 1950, 87:505.
34. Abernathy, R., The effect of cortisone on experimental brucellosis, *J. Clin. Invest.*, 1951, 30:626.
35. Schmidt, L. H., and W. L. Squires, The influence of cortisone on primate malaria, *J. Exp. Med.*, 1951, 94:501.
36. Redmond, W. B., Influence of cortisone on natural course of malaria in the pigeon, *Proc. Soc. Exp. Biol. & Med.*, 1952, 79:258.
37. Jarpa, A., M. Agosin, R. Christen, and A. V. Atias, Ensayos de quimio terapia de la erfermedad de Chagas experimental, VII: Cortisona y fosfato de pentaquina, *Bol. de Inform. Parasit. Chilenas*, 1951, 6:25.
38. Shwartzman, G., and A. Fisher, Alterations of experimental poliomyelitis infection in the Syrian hamster with the aid of cortisone, *J. Exp. Med.*, 1952, 95:347.
39. Selye, H., Further studies concerning the participation of the adrenal cortex in the pathogenesis of arthritis, *Brit. Med. J.*, 1949, 2:1129.
40. Mogabgab, W. J., and L. Thomas, The effects of cortisone on bacterial infection; Group A hemolytic streptococcal infection in rabbtis, *J. Lab. & Clin. Med.*, 1952, 39:271.
41. Ragan, C., E. L. Howes, C. M. Plotz, K. Meyer, and J. L. Blunt: Effect of cortisone on production of granulation tissue in rabbit, *Proc. Soc. Exp. Biol. & Med.*, 1949, 72:718.
42. Baker, B. L., and W. L. Whitaker, Interference with wound healing by local action of adrenocortical steroids, *Endocrinology*, 1950, 46:544.
43. Spain, D., N. Molomut, and A. Haber, The effect of cortisone on the formation of granulation tissue in mice. *Am. J. Path.*, 1950, 26:710.
44. Shapiro, R., B. Taylor, and M. Taubenhaus, Local effects of cortisone on granulation tissue and the role of denervation and ischemia, *Proc. Soc. Exp. Biol. & Med.*, 1951, 76:854.
45. Bangham, A. D., The effect of cortisone on wound healing, *Brit. J. Exp. Path.*, 1951, 32:77.
46. Upton, A. C., and W. C. Coon, Effects of cortisone and adrenocorticotropic hormone on wound healing in normal and scorbutic guinea pigs, *Proc. Soc. Exp. Biol. & Med.*, 1951, 77:153.
47. Michael, M., and C. M. Whorton, Delay of early inflammatory response by cortisone, *Proc. Soc. Exp. Biol. & Med.*, 1951, 76:754.
48. Moon, V. H., and G. A. Tershakovec, Influence of cortisone upon acute inflammation, *Proc. Soc. Exp. Biol. & Med.*, 1952, 79:63.
49. Menkin, V., Further studies on mechanism of increased capillary perme-

ability in inflammation with aid of cortisone and ACTH, *Proc. Soc. Exp. Biol. & Med.*, 1951, 77:592.
50. Menkin, V., Effect of adrenal cortex extract on capillary permeability, *Am. J. Physiol.*, 1940, 129:691.
51. Crepea, S. B., G. E. Magnin, and C. V. Seastone, Effect of ACTH and cortisone on phagocytosis, *Proc. Soc. Exp. Biol. & Med.*, 1951, 77:704.
52. Bjørneboe, M., E. E. Fischel, and H. C. Stoerk, The effect of cortisone and ACTH on the concentration of circulating antibody, *J. Exp. Med.*, 1951, 93:37.
53. Germuth, F. G., Jr., and B. Ottinger, Effect of 17-hydroxy-11-dehydrocorticosterone (compound E) and of ACTH on Arthus reaction and antibody formation in the rabbit, *Proc. Soc. Exp. Biol. & Med.*, 1950, 74:815.

    Germuth, F. G., Jr., J. Oyama, and B. Ottinger, The mechanism of action of 17-hydroxy-11-dehydrocorticosterone (compound E) of the adrenocorticotropic hormone in experimental hypersensitivity in rabbits, *J. Exp. Med.*, 1951, 94:139.
54. Fischel, E. E., Relationship of adrenal cortical activity to immune responses, *Bull. N.Y. Acad. Med.*, 1950, 26:255.

Chapter 11

THE EFFECT OF ACTH AND CORTISONE
UPON ALLERGIC DISEASES [1]

BY A. McGEHEE HARVEY, LAWRENCE E. SHULMAN, AND EDITH H.
SCHOENRICH, *The Department of Medicine, The Johns Hopkins
University School of Medicine*

IN THE HALF CENTURY which has elapsed since the classical studies of Von Pirquet on serum sickness, interest in the possible role of hypersensitivity in the pathogenesis of many human diseases has been widespread. It has been clearly recognized for many years that hypersensitivity in the human subject develops after repeated exposure not only to foreign protein but also to an ever-growing list of chemical substances which apparently combine with body proteins to form the antigenic complex. The resulting production of antibody sets the stage for the allergic inflammatory reaction which blossoms upon subsequent contact with the exciting antigen. The resulting manifestations vary from minor skin eruptions to severe and fatal reactions. Aside from the conditions which frequently occur, such as urticaria, angioneurotic edema, asthma, arthritis, lymphadenopathy, and fever, severe changes may occur, such as agranulocytosis, thrombocytopenia, and hemolytic anemia. One of the concepts to explain the broad spectrum of changes which may occur is that of the so-called "shock organ" which serves to categorize the various types of allergic reactions seen in human subjects, and a given antigen may in different sensitized individuals produce widely diverse reactions, such as urticaria, hay fever, asthma, purpura, or arthritis. What mechanisms determine these different responses in the host is not understood, but they may well determine the nature of the clinical picture in the patient who develops one of the diseases in which the prominent lesions are collagen and vascular tissue injury.

Various concepts have been put forth to explain the mechanism of the

[1] Part of the Cortisone and ACTH used in these experiments was purchased through a grant-in-aid from the Division of Research Grants and Fellowships, National Institute of Health, United States Public Health Service.

allergic inflammatory reaction. One postulates a direct injury to cells resulting from the union of antigen and antibody with the liberation of histamine, acetylcholine, or other physiologically active substances. Another envisages the inactivation of an enzyme inhibitor normally present resulting in the release of proteolytic enzyme activity, which in turn attacks the cells, freeing these physiologically active substances. Two different types of reaction may follow the application of antigen to the skin in the sensitive subject: one is the familiar "flare and wheal" reaction, which occurs immediately; the second is the delayed, or tuberculin, type reaction, in which the tissue response develops slowly and progressively and persists for several days (1). Numerous observers have now studied the effect of ACTH and cortisone in doses sufficient to induce a clinical remission in patients with allergic disease on the dermal reactivity to histamine and to various antigens. In most of these studies the skin was not the site of the disease process in these patients, although it did respond to the injection of suitable antigens. Studies have also been carried out on the effect of these hormones on the general vascular reactivity to histamine and the ability of the skin and adjacent tissues to liberate histamine-like substances after the administration of d-tubocurarine. The latter compound is one of several producing histamine-like effects after intracutaneous or intra-arterial injection attributable to the release of a histamine-like substance from the tissues (2). From these studies, it seems fairly clear that ACTH and cortisone do not affect the reactivity of the skin to histamine or the prompt reactivity to inhalent antigens, but they do diminish the delayed reactivity to bacterial antigens including tuberculin (3). Even a high level of adrenal-cortical stimulation produced by the intravenous administration of ACTH does not alter the ability of the skin and other tissues of the upper extremities to release histamine-like substance following the injection of d-tubocurarine or to respond to this substance or to histamine itself. These observations make it appear unlikely that the therapeutic effect of ACTH or cortisone in allergic diseases is mediated or accompanied by a general reduction in the reactivity to or availability of histamine. It is of interest that the antihistaminic compounds, which do influence the immediate skin reaction to antigens and also the reaction to histamine itself, fail to have a striking influence on such hypersensitive states as serum sickness and asthma, which are dramatically altered by the adrenal hormone. Of considerable importance would seem to be the fact that the delayed, or tuberculin type, of skin reaction may be very strikingly inhibited by raising the level of adrenal-cortical activity, while this type of reaction is not inhibited by antihistamine compounds. Further study of the differences between the prompt and delayed reactions to antigens may help to elucidate the mechanisms by which ACTH reduces the inflammatory response to a variety of stimuli.

It should be emphasized that the skin was not the site of allergic disease in the patients in whom dermal reactivity was studied, although the skin did respond to the injection of suitable antigens. Numerous clinical observations have shown that when the skin is the site of the allergic disease in patients with drug hypersensitivity the administration of ACTH and cortisone abolishes these cutaneous manifestations, such as giant urticaria, which are supposedly the counterpart of the prompt, or anaphylactic, type of sensitivity and the "wheal and flare" response to histamine. While these observations have involved different antigens from those employed in the studies just described and different routes of exposure in most instances, they do suggest that ACTH and cortisone diminish prompt dermal reactivity to antigens more readily when the skin itself is altered by the allergic disease. Again, an understanding of this difference might lead to important facts concerning the mechanism of action of ACTH and cortisone on the tissues and their response to disease.

Of further interest in this regard is the reaction which may occur from the application of certain alkaloids to the skin and mucous membranes. Irritation of the conjunctiva, lids, and adjacent cutaneous surfaces may develop during the course of local administration of atropine to the eye. Atropine apparently can combine with the protein in the tears to form stable salts to which a sensitivity develops. In the cases which have been treated with ACTH or cortisone there was no systemic hypersensitivity reaction, although the same type of eruption appeared in 24 to 48 hours after a cutaneous patch test in an uninvolved area with an ointment containing the alkaloid. Under adequate treatment with ACTH or cortisone there is a rapid healing of the skin lesions, and reaction to the patch test is essentially completely blocked. If hormonal treatment is continued, atropine may be reapplied without exciting any reaction (4).

ACTH and cortisone have been demonstrated to have a very dramatic effect in controlling the inflammatory and exudative phases of

ALLERGIC DISEASES

various diseases of the conjunctiva and uveal tract in which hypersensitivity is thought to play a role. Study of these diseases in the eye is of particular importance, for direct visual observations of the tissue changes may be made. This organ is likewise particularly suitable for experimental study. Nongranulomatous iritis is thought to represent a reaction due to bacterial hypersensitivity. In ocular tuberculosis the inflammatory reaction supposedly depends upon a sensitivity of the tissues to tuberculoprotein. Also, there is some evidence that sympathetic ophthalmia results from development of sensitivity to the patient's own uveal tract pigment. These hormones abolish the inflammatory phase of the disease in all of these situations. There are certain well-defined ocular allergic reactions in the rabbit, including the ophthalmic reaction to foreign protein and the focal reaction produced in tuberculous eyes by the systemic injection of tuberculin, which are particularly suitable for experimental study of the effect of ACTH and cortisone. If rabbits are suitably sensitized to horse serum by repeated intravenous injection and then given an anterior chamber inoculation of horse serum, a violent ocular reaction with conjunctivitis, iritis, and hypopyon results. This reaction develops after twenty-four hours and persists for ten to twelve days. It can be blocked by the previous administration of cortisone or ACTH. When normal rabbits are inoculated subcutaneously with a small amount of a six weeks old culture of human tubercle bacilli they run an asymptomatic course, and six weeks later they show cutaneous hypersensitivity to PPD. Three weeks later these animals are given an anterior chamber injection of a small number of tubercle bacilli. After another period of three weeks, all animals show evidence of a secondary ocular tuberculosis with slight pericorneal congestion and minute tubercles in the iris. If these immuno-allergic animals with early secondary ocular tuberculosis are given an injection of tuberculin systemically, the diseased eye responds in twenty-four hours with a violent inflammatory reaction. This reaction is completely suppressed in the cortisone-treated animal. If the animals are kept on cortisone an interesting phenomenon is observed. The basic inflammatory reaction associated with the tuberculosis is not present, but the tubercles in the iris continue to increase in size, presenting a picture of progressive nodular tuberculosis of the eye devoid of the usual inflammatory reaction (5). Although from these experiments it is quite clear that cortisone has the ability to block the inflammatory phase of the allergic reaction, further experiments have shown that a similar blocking effect may be seen when the inflammation is not related to hypersensitivity. It has been demonstrated that cortisone injections for several days prior to the anterior-chamber injection and for five days afterwards completely block the inflammatory reaction to the introduction of glycerin into the eye. The instillation of an infusion of jequirity seeds into the conjunctival sac produces a violent conjunctivitis. This inflammatory reaction can also be successfully blocked by ACTH or cortisone (6). Such experiments as these confirm the clinical observations that ACTH and cortisone have a dramatic effect on ocular inflammatory and exudative reactions. One cannot assume that these hormones inhibit or influence the antigen-antibody reaction, as the inflammatory reaction caused by irritants applied for the first time is blocked equally well. Experiments of this type in the eye may serve as a screening mechanism for comparing the value of other substances which may be thought to have a similar action to ACTH and cortisone. The eye would also seem to be a suitable place for studying in detail biochemical changes which occur in these various types of inflammatory reaction and the mechanism by which they are blocked when the level of circulating adrenal hormone is high.

The dramatic effects of ACTH and cortisone in suppressing the activity of the disease process in rheumatic fever, rheumatoid arthritis, disseminated lupus erythematosus, and periarteritis nodosa have been repeatedly demonstrated. Of interest is the fact that these diseases display a rather impressive group of phenomena known to occur as a part of the anaphylactic reaction in serum sickness, including sterile and migratory pulmonary consolidation of a characteristic type. Focal collagen degeneration of the anaphylactic type is well known in rheumatoid arthritis and is the basic lesion of the subcutaneous nodule seen in this disease. It is well known that a given antigen may produce in different individuals such widely divergent reactions as urticaria, asthma, purpura, and arthritis, manifestations which are seen during the course of certain of the above-mentioned diseases. Rich and others have shown that anatomical lesions similar to those seen in these so-called collagen vascular diseases can be produced in rabbits by anaphylactic hypersensitivity. It has been of considerable interest to observe that the production of these lesions can be inhibited by the administration of ACTH and cortisone. Rich and his colleagues have performed three separate experiments, comprising a total of 118 animals, all sensitized with horse serum in the same manner and half of them treated with either ACTH or cortisone. Of the 59 control animals, 51, or 86.4 percent, developed endocarditis, periarteritis nodosa, or both, while such lesions were found in only 23.6 percent of the animals treated with one of these hormones (7). This correlates well with the fact that healing of active periarteritis nodosa in the human subject can be demonstrated during the administration of ACTH or cortisone. Inhibition of the vascular injury induced by horse-serum hypersensitivity has been demonstrated in the living animal by Ebert and his coworkers, utilizing the rabbit-ear-chamber technique for observation of the tissues (8).

In the course of his experiments, using cortisone-treated rabbits, Rich found that many of the glomeruli showed a specific type of vascular lesion. These alterations consisted in focal aneurysmal-like dilatations of glomerular capillaries with rupture and hemorrhage or hyalinization of the contained blood or inspissated plasma, producing homogenous masses in the tufts. These hyaline masses resemble closely the isolated globular, hyalinized masses that occur in the glomeruli of certain patients with diabetes mellitus—the Kimmelstiel-Wilson lesion (9). Similar lesions have now been found in human subjects treated intensively with ACTH. These findings are of unusual interest in that they clearly demonstrate the production of a specific type of vascular lesion in the presence of excessive amounts of a naturally occurring hormonal substance.

Most of these observations which have been presented raise questions rather than answer them. Many impressive clinical phenomena have resulted from the administration of these hormones to patients with a wide variety of allergic diseases. Such clinical observations should provide the stimulus for experimental studies which may further clarify understanding of the hypersensitive state and its relations to naturally occurring disease, as well as to a better understanding of the mechanism of action of the hormones themselves.

REFERENCES

1. Harvey, A. M., Introduction to series of papers on studies on ACTH and cortisone, *Bull. Johns Hopkins Hosp.*, 1951, 87:349.
2. Grob, D., E. H. Schoenrich, W. L. Winkenwerder, and A. M. Harvey, The influence of ACTH on the reactivity of the bronchial tree, skin, and

secretory glands to specific antigens, histamine and mecholyl in bronchial asthma. Proc. 2d ACTH Conference, 1951, I, 499.
3. Long, J. B., and C. B. Favour, The ability of ACTH and cortisone to alter delayed type bacterial hypersensitivity, *Bull. Johns Hopkins Hosp.*, 1950, 87:186.
4. Carey, R. A., A. M. Harvey, J. E. Howard, and P. F. Wagley, The effect of adrenocorticotropic hormone (ACTH) and cortisone on drug hypersensitivity reactions, *Bull. Johns Hopkins Hosp.*, 1950, 87:354.
5. Woods, A. C., and R. M. Wood, The action of ACTH and cortisone on experimental ocular inflammation, *Bull. Johns Hopkins Hosp.*, 1950, 87:482.
6. ―――― The effect of cortisone and ACTH on ocular inflammation secondary to injection of irritant substances, *Bull. Johns Hopkins Hosp.*, 1952, 90:134.
7. Rich, A. R., M. Berthrong, and I. L. Bennett, Jr., The effect of cortisone upon the experimental cardiovascular and renal lesions produced by anaphylactic hypersensitivity, *Bull. Johns Hopkins Hosp.*, 1950, 87:257.
8. Ebert, R. H., and R. W. Wissler, Studies on the pathogenesis of serum sickness using the ear chamber technique, with preliminary results of cortisone treatment, *J. Lab. & Clin. Med.*, 1950, 36:818.
9. Rich, A. R., M. Berthrong, I. L. Bennett, Jr., T. H. Cochran, P. C. Griffith, and D. C. McGoon, The effect of ACTH and cortisone upon experimental glomerulonephritis, *Trans. Assn. Am. Phys.*, 1951, 54:257.

Chapter 12

THE EFFECTS OF CORTISONE ON BACTERIAL
INFECTION AND INTOXICATION [1]

By LEWIS THOMAS, *Professor of Pediatrics and Medicine, American Legion Memorial Research Professor, University of Minnesota Medical School, Minneapolis*

WE ARE CONCERNED in this paper with an account of two sets of experiments dealing with two separate and apparently unrelated effects of cortisone in the rabbit—first, the production of susceptibility to lethal infection by living microorganisms, in this case group A hemolytic streptococci, and second, the production of susceptibility to necrotizing vascular damage by certain bacterial toxins, in this case the toxins of meningococci and S. *marcescens*. In addition, a third set of experiments will be described, which provides evidence that these two effects of cortisone may be based on the same underlying mechanism.

First, let us consider the effect of cortisone on streptococcal infection (1). When normal rabbits are given an injection of living group A hemolytic streptococci into the skin, there is an intense local inflammatory reaction at the injected site, which becomes visible within approximately eight hours. The affair usually ends with the skin infection, and the animals do not usually develop positive blood cultures or exhibit other evidences of systemic infection.

Treatment with cortisone for three or four days before skin infection, by giving a daily dose of 5 mg or more per kilo, causes a marked alteration in this response to streptococci. The local reaction is greatly minimized, and often there is no visible inflammation on the following day. At this time, however, blood cultures become positive in most rabbits, and when cortisone is continued the majority of animals die with overwhelming septicemia within three to ten days after inoculation.

The outcome in a series of typical experiments is illustrated in Table 1. Here it will be seen that in a group of sixty-six rabbits treated with cortisone, septicemia occurred in sixty-four, and death in fifty-eight.

[1] From the Pediatric Research Laboratories, Heart Hospital, University of Minnesota Medical School, Minneapolis.

In contrast, in a group of sixty control rabbits infected with the same inocula of streptococci without cortisone, only eight developed septicemia, and only five died.

ACTH, in a dosage of 5 mg every six hours, had a similar effect on streptococcal infection, as is illustrated in Table 1.

TABLE 1

THE EFFECT OF CORTISONE AND ACTH ON THE RESPONSE TO INTRADERMAL INFECTION BY GROUP A STREPTOCOCCI IN RABBITS

Treatment	Number of Rabbits	Number Having Bacteremia	Number Dead
Cortisone [a]	66	64	58
None	60	8	5
ACTH [b]	8	7	7
None	8	0	0

[a] Cortisone given daily in dose of 5 mg per kilo, beginning three days before infection.
[b] ACTH given in dose of 5 mg per kilo 4 times daily, beginning one day before infection.

The extent of septicemia in the cortisone-treated animals, as judged by colony counts of the blood cultures, was remarkably at variance with the general appearance of the animals. Until a few hours before death, and sometimes until the moment of death, the rabbits appeared to be in reasonably good health, despite the presence of many thousands of streptococci per ml in their blood.

Equally remarkable was the absence of evidence of tissue damage in these animals, either by gross or by microscopic inspection of the organs. The most striking histological change was in the heart, and here the tissues were not damaged, nor was there even tissue reaction, but there was extensive streptococcal proliferation, as is shown in Figure 1. This heart was placed in fixative immediately after death, and it may therefore be assumed that the colony-like aggregations of cocci were present among the muscle fibers during life.

The effect of cortisone could be prevented by treatment with penicillin, provided that it was begun within the first three days after infection and given in extremely large doses. Desoxycorticosterone and additional salt in the diet, which have been reported to antagonize other actions of cortisone, had no effect on the enhancement of infection by cortisone. The same was true of pituitary somatotropic hormone, which had no effect on septicemia or mortality when given daily in doses of 10 mg per kilo (2).

Our studies of the effect of cortisone on the response to bacterial toxin began as a series of relatively simple experiments designed to determine whether cortisone would inhibit the Shwartzman reaction. The answer which was obtained was unequivocally negative, but certain

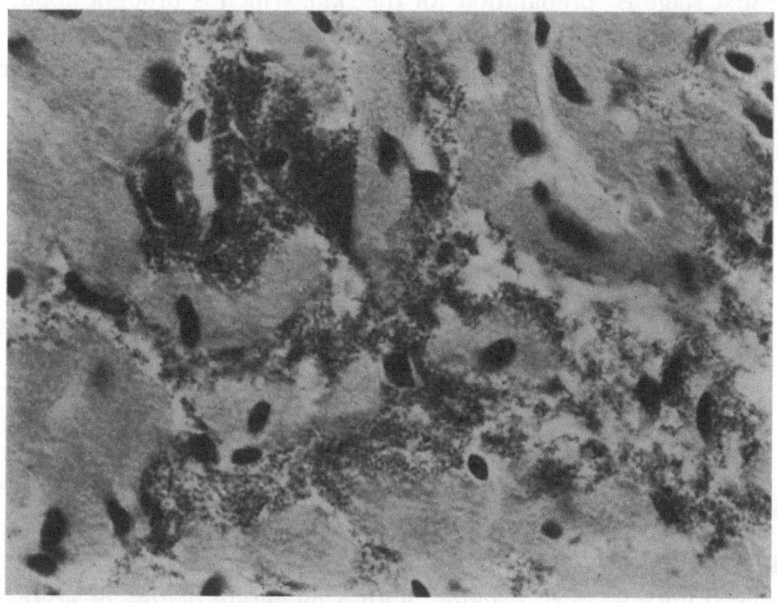

FIGURE 1. SECTION OF MYOCARDIUM FROM A CORTISONE-TREATED RABBIT INFECTED WITH GROUP A STREPTOCOCCI AND SACRIFICED THREE DAYS AFTER INFECTION

observations were made in the course of these experiments which may have bearing on the mechanism of the Shwartzman reaction itself. These observations, reported in detail elsewhere (3, 4), may be summarized as follows:

First, cortisone in doses of 25 mg or more per kilo per day, with a pretreatment period of three days, did not inhibit the local Shwartzman reaction. This is shown in Table 2, in which it may be seen that the Shwartzman reaction occurred in the same proportion of treated and untreated rabbits. The intensity and extent of the skin reactions were the same in the animals which received cortisone as in those which did not. Similar results were obtained with ACTH, in a dosage of 10 mg every six hours, following a pretreatment period of two days. In fact, the Shwartzman reaction occurred more rapidly and with greater intensity in the ACTH-treated rabbits than in the untreated controls.

It was next observed that cortisone produced an effect which seemed to be the equivalent of one phase of the Shwartzman reaction. It will be recalled that the Shwartzman reaction involves two separate stages (5). The first stage is "preparation" of the skin, which is brought about by the intradermal injection of toxin from a variety of gram-negative organisms. An optimal period of eighteen to twenty-four hours is required for preparation to take place. During this time the skin shows a vigor-

TABLE 2

THE EFFECT OF CORTISONE AND ACTH ON THE DERMAL SHWARTZMAN REACTION

Treatment	Bacterial Toxin	Number of Rabbits	Number Having Positive Reactions
Cortisone [a]	Meningococcal	6	6
	S. marcescens	10	9
ACTH [b]	Meningococcal	6	6
None	Meningococcal	6	6
	S. marcescens	10	9

[a] Cortisone given in a dose of 25 mg per kilo, beginning three days before preparation.

[b] ACTH given in dose of 10 mg per kilo 4 times daily, beginning two days before preparation.

ous local inflammatory reaction, with a moderate degree of erythema and edema. The second stage is "provocation" of the reaction, and this is accomplished by an intravenous injection of small amounts of the same or other bacterial toxins. Within two to three hours after the intravenous provocation, the prepared skin area exhibits multiple petechial hemorrhages which rapidly coalesce, and hemorrhagic necrosis of the skin is the final result.

In cortisone-treated rabbits, the first stage of this reaction was very different. Instead of edema and erythema, the injected skin site showed no visible reaction during the first twelve hours. After about twenty hours the area became somewhat pale, and then numerous small petechiae appeared. Usually these remained discrete, although sometimes they coalesced and presented an appearance strongly resembling a mild Shwartzman reaction.

Histologically, the skin tissue showed much less inflammatory cell

BACTERIAL INFECTION AND INTOXICATION

infiltration than is seen in the prepared skin of normal rabbits. In addition, there were many areas in which the small vessels appeared to be occluded by leukocyte-platelet thrombi, a lesion which has been shown by Stetson (6) to be a characteristic feature of the developing Shwartzman reaction after the intravenous injection of toxin. In the prepared skin of normal rabbits such thrombi were not seen.

It was shown by Becker (7) and by Stetson and Good (8) that the dermal Shwartzman reaction is completely prevented by nitrogen mustard when this drug is given three days prior to provocation of the reaction. We have found that the primary hemorrhagic skin reaction to toxin in cortisone-treated rabbits is also completely prevented by nitrogen mustard (4).

The systemic counterpart of the local Shwartzman reaction is the so-called generalized Shwartzman reaction. It is produced by giving both the first, or preparing, injection and the second, or provoking, injection by the intravenous route. The characteristic pathological lesion of the reaction is bilateral cortical necrosis of the kidneys. This lesion is illustrated in Figure 2, which shows the kidney of a rabbit which received

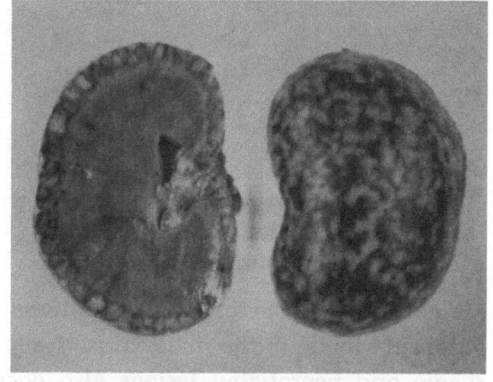

FIGURE 2. KIDNEY OF A RABBIT WITH THE GENERALIZED SHWARTZMAN REACTION PRODUCED BY TWO INTRAVENOUS INJECTIONS OF MENINGOCOCCAL TOXIN

two intravenous injections of meningococcal toxin spaced twenty-four hours apart. As in the dermal Shwartzman reaction, it is essential that two injections be given and that there be a suitable time interval between the injections. A single intravenous injection of toxin does not produce this reaction in normal rabbits, even when the amount of toxin is many times greater than the amount required to produce renal necrosis when given in two divided doses. The only circumstance in which a single injection of toxin has been reported to cause the generalized

Shwartzman reaction in rabbits is in pregnancy (9), which is of particular interest in the light of the observations to be described.

In all of the kidneys with this lesion, the glomeruli, as shown in Figure 3, contain extensive masses of homogeneous eosinophilic material within the glomerular capillaries. This material appears very early in the reaction, before there is any gross evidence of cortical necrosis. Its nature is not known. It does not appear to contain formed elements,

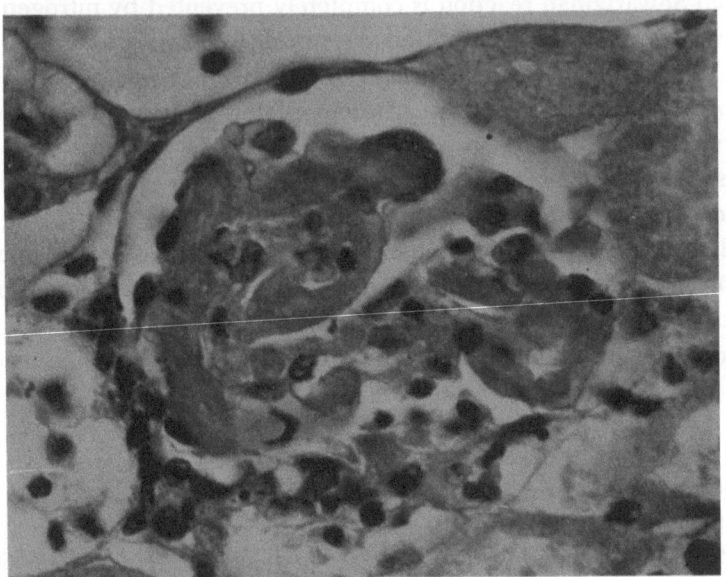

FIGURE 3. GLOMERULUS OF KIDNEY WITH EARLY BILATERAL CORTICAL NECROSIS, SHOWING HOMOGENEOUS MATERIAL OCCLUDING THE CAPILLARIES

platelets, or leukocytes. In preparations stained by the Hotchkiss periodic acid method, the material is strongly Schiff positive (4). Hemorrhagic and necrotizing lesions also occur in other organs, including lungs, liver, spleen, and the gastrointestinal tract.

This, then, is the generalized Shwartzman reaction, produced by two intravenous injections of toxin. As we have already seen, an intradermal injection of toxin in cortisone-treated rabbits causes a "primary" hemorrhagic skin lesion resembling the local Shwartzman reaction. It was obviously important to determine what effect a single intravenous injection of toxin would have in rabbits pretreated for three days with cortisone.

BACTERIAL INFECTION AND INTOXICATION

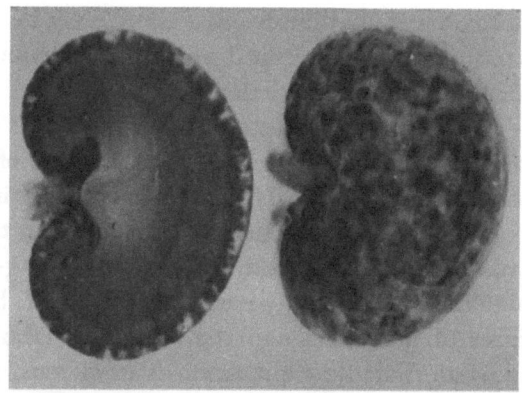

FIGURE 4. KIDNEY OF A CORTISONE-TREATED RABBIT WHICH RECEIVED A SINGLE INTRAVENOUS INJECTION OF MENINGOCOCCAL TOXIN, SHOWING BILATERAL CORTICAL NECROSIS

The result is illustrated in Figure 4, which shows the kidney of a cortisone-treated rabbit which died within thirty hours after a single intravenous injection of meningococcal toxin; the lesion is bilateral renal cortical necrosis. Identical renal lesions were produced by a single intravenous injection of S. *marcescens* toxin in cortisone-treated rabbits, with an incidence of approximately 70 percent, as is illustrated in Table 3. In its gross and microscopic appearance, including the same deposits of homogeneous, eosinophilic, Schiff-positive material within glomerular capillaries, the lesion was indistinguishable from the renal lesion of the generalized Shwartzman reaction. In addition to the renal lesion, similar hemorrhagic and necrotizing lesions occurred in lungs, liver, spleen, and intestines.

The generalized Shwartzman reaction produced by two injections of toxin and the reaction in cortisone-treated rabbits given one injection

TABLE 3

THE PRODUCTION OF BILATERAL RENAL CORTICAL NECROSIS IN CORTISONE-TREATED RABBITS BY A SINGLE INJECTION OF BACTERIAL TOXIN

Experimental Procedure	Number of Rabbits	Number Having Bilateral Renal Cortical Necrosis
25 mg cortisone daily for 4 days; 0.4 mg S. *marcescens* toxin i.v. on 3d day	100	70
25 mg cortisone daily for 4 days; no toxin	50	0
0.4 mg S. *marcescens* toxin i.v.; no cortisone	150	0

of toxin were both prevented completely by nitrogen mustard, with the same dosage of mustard which was previously shown to prevent the local Shwartzman reaction (4).

In attempting to account for these effects of cortisone, several possibilities were considered. The first, in view of the known effect of cortisone on infection (10), was that systemic infection by other bacteria may have been activated by cortisone, thus taking the place of the provoking stimulus for both the local and the generalized Shwartzman reactions. This cannot be entirely excluded, but repeated negative cultures of the blood and the tissues of rabbits with positive reactions indicate that the explanation is erroneous. Another possibility is that the cortisone-treated animals may have a reduced capacity to localize toxin or to remove it from the blood, with the result that the vascular bed is exposed to recirculating toxin for a longer time than in normal rabbits.

One indirect approach to this was to study the effect of cortisone on the retention of toxin in the skin. It is known that in normal rabbits the bacterial toxins employed for the Shwartzman reaction are absorbed only to a small extent, if at all, when injected into the skin. Animals show no evidences of systemic intoxication following intradermal injections of amounts of toxin which would be rapidly lethal if given by vein. Moreover, neither the local nor the generalized Shwartzman reaction can be elicited when the second, or provoking, injection is given intradermally instead of intravenously.

This capacity to retain toxin in the skin is lacking in the cortisone-treated rabbit, and the end result of an intradermal injection of toxin is the same as if the toxin were given by vein. The experiment shown in Table 4 illustrates this finding. In the first group are eight rabbits treated with cortisone and injected intradermally with prodigiosus toxin in a dose of 0.4 mg, the amount of toxin which is required for the consistent production of renal necrosis when given intravenously. Seven of the eight developed bilateral cortical necrosis of the kidneys. The second group showed the conventional generalized Shwartzman reaction, with two intravenous injections of the same amount of toxin in normal rabbits; all of these animals developed renal necrosis. In the third group, also without cortisone, it is shown that the reaction does not occur when the animals are prepared by an intravenous injection and then given the same amount of toxin intradermally.

These observations indicate that sufficient absorption of toxin from the skin occurred in the cortisone-treated rabbits to produce the kidney lesion of the generalized Shwartzman reaction. Since the dose of toxin was the same as the amount required by the intravenous route, it can be assumed that a considerable proportion of the toxin was absorbed.

TABLE 4

BILATERAL RENAL CORTICAL NECROSIS AFTER A SINGLE INTRADERMAL INJECTION OF S. MARCESCENS TOXIN IN CORTISONE-TREATED RABBITS

Experimental Procedure	Number of Rabbits	Number Having Bilateral Renal Cortical Necrosis
25 mg cortisone daily for 4 days, 0.4 mg S. marcescens toxin intradermally on 3d day	8	7
2 i.v. injections of 0.4 mg S. marcescens toxin, 24 hours apart; no cortisone	4	4
0.4 mg S. marcescens toxin i.v., followed 24 hours later by 0.4 mg intradermally; no cortisone	4	0

It seemed possible that a comparable protective mechanism involving internal tissues, a mechanism normally responsible for the removal or fixation of toxin circulating in the blood, might be similarly impaired by cortisone, thus allowing toxin to circulate for a longer time or to act on tissues which are normally protected.

One protective mechanism which seems to be involved in the reaction to this class of toxins is the reticulo-endothelial cell system. Beeson (11) has shown that blockade of these cells by thorotrast or trypan blue results in an increased susceptibility to the dermal Shwartzman reaction. Also, the marked vulnerability of lymphoid tissues to hemorrhagic necrosis in the local and generalized Shwartzman reactions suggests that localization of toxin may occur in such tissues. And finally, it is known that cortisone causes dissolution and atrophy of lymphoid tissue, presumably a source from which reticulo-endothelial cells may be derived, and if such cells are involved in defense against bacterial toxin one might expect to see increased vulnerability in cortisone-treated animals.

With this in mind, the following working hypothesis was formulated for testing: The vascular necrosis which characterizes the generalized Shwartzman reaction results from the action of bacterial toxin. In normal animals this kind of tissue damage is prevented by the efficient functioning of the reticulo-endothelial cells, which remove or fix such toxins. When these cells are unable to function properly, an intravenous injection of toxin will produce generalized damage to blood vessels. This state of affairs is created in the generalized Shwartzman reaction by the first, or preparing, intravenous injection of toxin, which is taken up by this system of cells and alters their function so that they are unable to interfere with a second intravenous injection of toxin twenty-four hours later.

If this is the correct supposition, it should be possible to create the same experimental conditions by interfering in other ways with the function of the reticulo-endothelial cells. Thorotrast and trypan blue have both been shown to be taken up by these cells, and both of these colloidal materials have been employed for "blockading" the RE system. Accordingly, the following experiment was performed. Rabbits were given an intravenous injection of bacterial toxin at varying periods before and after an injection of thorotrast or trypan blue. The results were clear-cut (12). When the toxin was given six hours after thorotrast, or after trypan blue, the generalized Shwartzman reaction with bilateral cortical necrosis of the kidneys occurred in all animals, except for those which died within too short a time after the injection of the toxin for the gross lesions to develop. Table 5 shows the incidence of renal necrosis and death in rabbits given varying amounts of meningococcal toxin six hours after an injection of thorotrast, compared with the results obtained with the same doses of toxin without thorotrast. It may be seen that the lethal effect of toxin was tremendously enhanced by thorotrast. By itself, thorotrast caused no deaths or renal lesions.

Another point of resemblance between the effect of thorotrast and that of cortisone was in the reaction to toxin injected into the skin. It will be recalled that the cortisone-treated rabbits developed petechial hemorrhages in the injected skin area, and also showed evidence of sufficient absorption of toxin from the skin to produce bilateral cortical necrosis of the kidneys. Similar events occurred after a single intra-

TABLE 5

BILATERAL RENAL CORTICAL NECROSIS AND DEATH IN RABBITS GIVEN A SINGLE INTRAVENOUS INJECTION OF MENINGOCOCCAL TOXIN SIX HOURS AFTER AN INJECTION OF THOROTRAST

DILUTION OF TOXIN [a]	THOROTRAST 6 HOURS BEFORE TOXIN			NO THOROTRAST		
	Number of Rabbits	Number Dead	Number Having Bilateral Renal Cortical Necrosis	Number of Rabbits	Number Dead	Number Having Bilateral Renal Cortical Necrosis
1–20	9	9	0	10	1	0
1–80	9	9	2	6	0	0
1–320	9	9	6	12	0	0
1–1280	6	6	5	4	0	0
1–5120	6	3	4	4	0	0
1–10,000	6	0	3	4	0	0
1–50,000	4	0	0	4	0	0
No toxin	10	0	0	0	0	0

[a] Thorotrast (Heyden Chemical Corp.) given in dose of 3 cc per kilo, intravenously.

dermal injection of toxin in thorotrast-treated rabbits—namely, petechiae appeared in the skin on the following day, and the animals died with renal cortical necrosis.

It is obvious that thorotrast and trypan blue may have many other biological effects aside from their action on reticulo-endothelial cells, and this phenomenon may be due to some mechanism other than blockade. A point in favor of its being blockade is that when the order of injections was reversed and thorotrast was given a few hours *after* toxin, instead of before, the animals did not become ill, and the kidneys remained normal (12).

We have suggested that the effect of cortisone on the response to a single injection of toxin may be imitated by interference with the reticulo-endothelial system by toxin itself, or by blockade with thorotrast. The hypothesis would be strengthened if it could be shown that the other effect of cortisone described in this paper—the enhancement of streptococcal infection—could also be imitated in this fashion.

To test this, rabbits were injected intravenously with thorotrast and six hours later were given an injection of streptococci in the skin. It will be recalled that in cortisone-treated rabbits the local skin reaction to streptococcal infection is markedly diminished and that the animals regularly develop streptococcal septicemia. Similar minimal skin reactions accompanied by positive blood cultures occurred in the thorotrast-treated rabbits. Moreover, the lethal effect of streptococcal infection was greatly enhanced by thorotrast, when streptococci were injected intravenously after an injection of thorotrast. These events are illustrated in Table 6.

TABLE 6

THE EFFECT OF THOROTRAST ON THE RESPONSE TO INFECTION BY GROUP A STREPTOCOCCI IN RABBITS

Experimental Procedure	Number of Rabbits	Number Dead
Intravenous thorotrast followed by intravenous streptococci 6 hours later	10	10
Intravenous streptococci; no thorotrast	10	1
Intravenous thorotrast; no streptococci	10	0

On the basis of these observations, there is reason to suspect that toxin, thorotrast, and streptococci may each be taken up by the same defense cell system. We have implied that competition for these cells may exist between thorotrast and toxin, and between thorotrast and streptococci. The next question is whether competition of the same sort can be demonstrated between toxin and streptococci.

First, we studied the effect of streptococci following the injection of toxin. When a systemic infection was produced by an intravenous injection of streptococci and this was followed after twenty-four hours or longer by an intravenous injection of meningococcal or *S. marcescens* toxin, a violent form of the generalized Shwartzman reaction occurred (13). The kidneys showed bilateral cortical necrosis, and many hemorrhages appeared in other tissues, including heart, lungs, and spleen. With adequate doses of streptococci and toxin, this reaction could be produced in more than 75 percent of the animals.

When the order was reversed, the streptococci being injected some hours after, instead of before, the toxin, the reaction was entirely different. Instead of developing the generalized Shwartzman reaction, these animals developed overwhelming streptococcal septicemia similar to that observed in the animals given thorotrast or cortisone, and at autopsy no hemorrhagic or necrotizing lesions were present in the kidneys or other organs. The incidence of septicemia and death in a group of rabbits given streptococci after toxin is shown in Table 7.

Summary.—Two apparently separate effects of cortisone have been described: first, the effect on susceptibility to infection by Group A hemolytic streptococci, resulting in lethal septicemia; and secondly, the effect on the susceptibility to vascular damage by bacterial toxins, resulting in lesions resembling the generalized Shwartzman reaction.

TABLE 7

THE EFFECT OF AN INTRAVENOUS INJECTION OF MENINGOCOCCAL TOXIN ON THE RESPONSE TO A SUBSEQUENT INJECTION OF GROUP A STREPTOCOCCI

Experimental Procedure	Number of Rabbits	Number Dead
Intravenous meningococcal toxin, followed by intravenous streptococci 12 hours later	9	8
Intravenous meningococcal toxin; no streptococci	6	0
Intravenous streptococci; no toxin	6	0

In an attempt to account for these effects, a working hypothesis has been set up in which it is suggested that cells of the reticulo-endothelial system are implicated in defense against both streptococcal infection and bacterial toxin. The effects of cortisone, it is suggested, are due to interference with the normal functioning of this system of cells.

In support of this hypothesis, it has been shown that reticulo-endothelial blockade by thorotrast, or by trypan blue, creates a state of affairs which is comparable to that produced by cortisone. A single injection of toxin produces the vascular lesions of the generalized Shwartzman reaction, and an injection of streptococci results in septicemia and death.

It is suggested that an effect which is analogous to that of cortisone may account for the occurrence of the generalized Shwartzman reaction when a streptococcal infection is followed by an injection of bacterial toxin, as well as for the occurrence of lethal septicemia when the order of injection is reversed and streptococci are given following a toxin injection. These events may result from the ability of each of these agents to interfere, during a crucial period of time, with the capacity of the reticulo-endothelial cells to defend the host against the other.

As an experimental model, this has much to offer in the study of certain complex disease states in which more than one infectious agent or toxic substance may be involved.

REFERENCES

1. Mogabgab, W. J., and L. Thomas, The effects of cortisone on bacterial infection, *J. Lab. & Clin. Med.*, 1952, 39:271.
2. Unpublished observations.
3. Thomas, L., and W. J. Mogabgab, Hemorrhagic skin lesions produced by intradermal meningococcus toxin in rabbits following treatment with ACTH or cortisone, *Proc. Soc. Exp. Biol. & Med.*, 1950, 74:829.
4. Thomas, L., and R. A. Good, The production of lesions resembling the dermal and generalized Shwartzman reaction by a single injection of bacterial toxin in cortisone-treated rabbits, *J. Exp. Med.*, 1952, 95:409.
5. Shwartzman, G., Phenomenon of Local Tissue Reactivity and Its Immunological, Pathological and Clinical Significance (Paul Hoeber, New York, 1937).
6. Stetson, C. A., Studies on the mechanism of the Shwartzman phenomenon; certain factors involved in the production of the local hemorrhagic necrosis, *J. Exp. Med.*, 1951, 93:489.
7. Becker, R. M., Suppression of local tissue reactivity, Shwartzman phenomenon, by nitrogen mustard, benzol, and X-ray irradiation, *Proc. Soc. Exp. Biol. & Med.*, 1948, 69:247.
8. Stetson, C. A., and R. A. Good, Studies on the mechanism of the Shwartzman phenomenon; evidence for the participation of polymorphonuclear leucocytes in the phenomenon, *J. Exp. Med.*, 1951, 93:49.
9. Apitz, K., A study of the generalized Shwartzman phenomenon, *J. Immunol.*, 1935, 29:255.
10. Thomas, L., Effect of cortisone and adrenocortocotropic hormone on infection, *Ann. Rev. Med.*, 1952, 3:1.
11. Beeson, P. B., Effect of reticulo-endothelial blockade on immunity to the Shwartzman phenomenon, *Proc. Soc. Exp. Biol. & Med.*, 1947, 64:146.
12. Good, R. A., and L. Thomas, Studies on the generalized Shwartzman reaction II, *J. Exp. Med.*, 1952, 96:625.
13. Thomas, L., F. W. Denny, Jr., and J. Floyd, Carditis in the generalized Shwartzman reaction produced with group A streptococci, *Fed. Proc.*, 1952, 11:484.

Chapter 13

OBSERVATIONS ON ADRENAL CORTICAL HORMONES IN PNEUMOCOCCAL AND INFLUENZA VIRAL INFECTIONS AND IN MALARIA [1]

By EDWARD H. KASS, *Senior Fellow in Virus Diseases of the National Research Council*, QUENTIN M. GEIMAN, AND MAXWELL FINLAND

THE INITIAL STUDIES on the effects of adrenocorticotropic hormone (ACTH) on lobar and viral pneumonias in man (1-2) are summarized in Figure 1, which shows what happened when a patient with type 8 pneumococcal pneumonia was given ACTH without antibiotics. This patient, and others so treated, underwent rapid defervescence following institution of therapy, with striking relief of symptoms and of such evidences of toxicity as malaise, anorexia, and lassitude. However, pneumococci persisted for weeks in the sputum and throat cultures, and bacteremia was demonstrated more than twenty-four hours after the patient was entirely afebrile and asymptomatic. In another patient (Figure 2), spread of the pneumonia to other lobes was observed during hormone therapy, while the patient was asymptomatic; this patient subsequently developed empyema.

Naturally, such striking dissociation of the clinical response from the bacteriologic status prompted further investigation. Several explanations for this paradoxical effect were suggested. The possibility that ACTH causes release of antibodies was largely ruled out when it was demonstrated that these patients showed no increase in circulating antibodies following administration of hormones; specific agglutinins and mouse protective antibodies appeared at the time when they would have been expected in the normal course of these infections.

In mice ACTH did not confer any increased capacity to survive ex-

[1] From the Thorndike Memorial Laboratory, Second and Fourth Medical Services (Harvard), Boston City Hospital, the Department of Medicine, Harvard Medical School, and the Department of Tropical Public Health, Harvard School of Public Health, Boston, Massachusetts; aided by a grant from the United States Public Health Service.

perimental pneumococcal infection; this was true even when the animals were partially protected by the prior administration of antibody (3). Indeed, infected mice treated with cortisone died sooner than the infected untreated controls, and the protective action of the antibody was diminished significantly.

In the case of influenza A infections (3), to which some immunity exists in adult mice, the lethal dose of virus was decreased by treatment of the mice with cortisone. ACTH, however, did not alter the lethal titer significantly even when used in very large doses. Neither hormone altered appreciably the rate of multiplication of the virus in the host

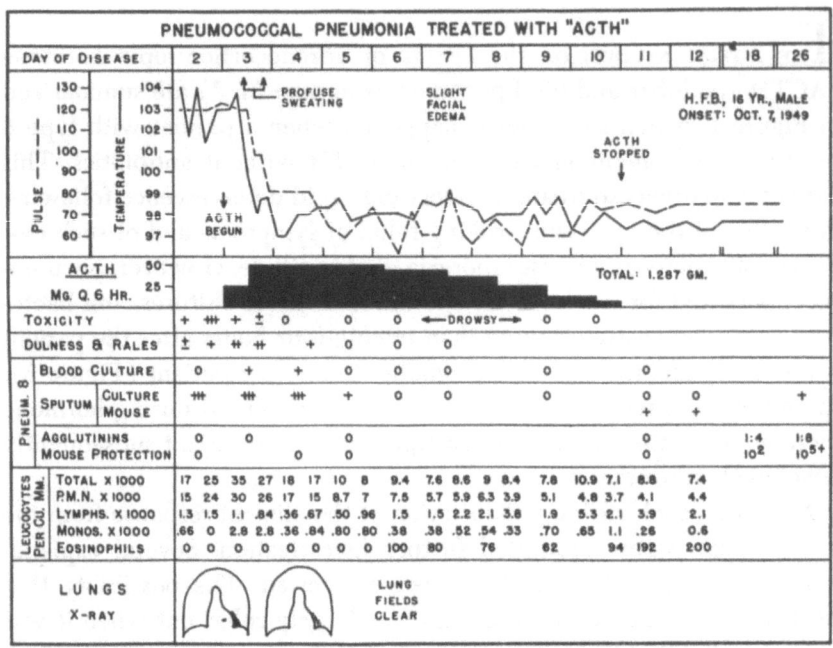

FIGURE 1. PNEUMOCOCCAL PNEUMONIA TREATED WITH "ACTH"
From Kass, Ingbar, and Finland (2)

lung, nor did they affect the maximum concentration of virus in the lungs. Other workers (4) have demonstrated a slightly unfavorable effect of ACTH on mortality in mice infected with influenza viruses, with no significant difference in the viral content of lungs of hormone-treated animals and untreated controls. The deleterious effect of the hormones must have been exerted, not so much on factors which inhibit

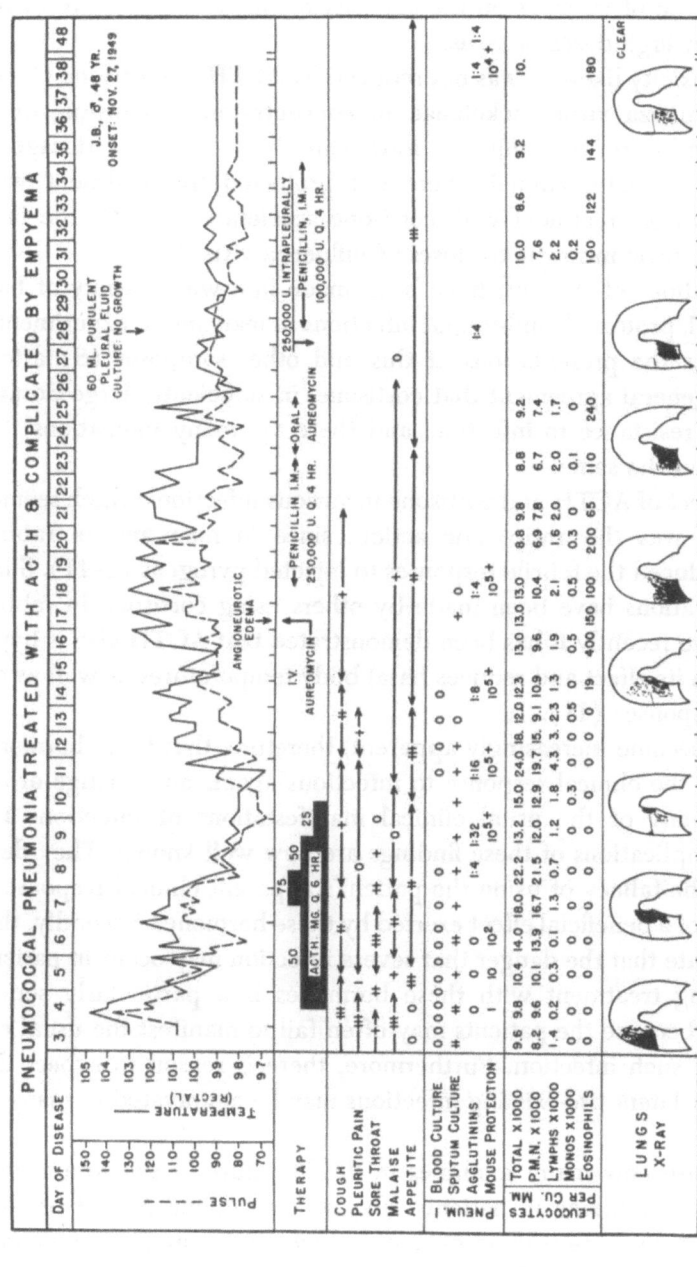

FIGURE 2. PNEUMOCOCCAL PNEUMONIA TREATED WITH ACTH AND COMPLICATED BY EMPYEMA
From Kass, Ingbar, and Finland (2)

multiplication of virus, as on the capacity of the host to survive in the presence of high doses of virus.

Acute toxicity likewise was not reduced by ACTH or cortisone (5–6). When influenza virus, rickettsiae in concentrated suspension, or S. *typhosa* endotoxin was injected intravenously in sufficient dosage to cause acute death, animals were not protected by treatment with ACTH, and pretreatment with cortisone accelerated slightly the fatal reaction to toxic intravenous doses of influenza virus (7).

Observations of this sort have been made in a wide variety of bacterial, viral, protozoal, and fungal infections in man and in experimental animals, as the presentations at this and other symposia (8) attest. There is general agreement that cortisone, in sufficiently large dosage, depresses resistance to infection, and there are many indications that ACTH does the same.

One effect of ACTH and cortisone in various infections which seemed consistent was the antipyretic action, since in man and in rabbits ACTH reduced the febrile responses to injected pyrogens (9–11). Similar observations have been made by others using cortisone in rabbits (12). More recently it has been demonstrated that ACTH also is hypothermic in its effect and reduces basal body temperatures as well as the febrile responses (11).

It has become increasingly apparent, therefore, that these hormones may alter the clinical response to infectious agents and change or obliterate many of the usual clinical manifestations of infection. The clinical implications of these findings are now well known. They demonstrate the fallacy of using the patient's apparent clinical response as evidence of a beneficial effect exerted by these hormones. Secondly, they demonstrate that the danger that severe infection may occur in patients undergoing treatment with these hormones is a particularly serious problem, because the patients may often fail to manifest the usual evidences of such infection. Furthermore, there is reason to expect that chronic or latent pre-existing infections may be aggravated in many instances.

There are now many examples in the literature of severe and even fatal sepsis occurring in patients who were receiving ACTH or cortisone in whom there was no evidence clinically to suggest infection of such severity (13–16). There is also evidence of dissemination of tuberculous infection in patients receiving ACTH or cortisone, and in some instances this has occurred in the absence of previous clinical evidence of the presence of any active tuberculosis (17). There are clear indications, experimentally, that organisms which are not usually fatal for certain hosts may become rapidly invasive and produce fatalities when the host animals are receiving one of these hormones (18–19).

Metabolic studies were instituted to determine whether during a severe infection, such as lobar pneumonia, some of the changes induced by the infection could be reversed by ACTH. The urinary excretion of various metabolites during the administration of ACTH to patients with lobar pneumonia was compared with the patterns of excretion during a twelve to eighteen hour control period. The patterns of excretion of electrolytes, phosphate, uric acid, and creatinine were consistent with changes which occur in the healthy individual receiving ACTH, and they were also consistent with the changes which have been observed in many inflammatory, neoplastic, and degenerative disorders studied in the same manner.

Four patients suffering from pneumonia were studied to determine the metabolic patterns in the acute disease unaffected by the administration of ACTH or cortisone (7). These patients were treated with penicillin, commencing 12–18 hours after admission, and were given weighed diets and 8–10 grams of sodium chloride daily. Acute studies of this type under adequate control are difficult to perform and to evaluate, but the data obtained indicated that during the acute phase of the illness there were striking losses of potassium and nitrogen, with retention of sodium and chloride. The potassium deficiency could not be explained on the basis of nitrogen loss alone. At the same time the excretion of corticoids and 17-ketosteroids was increased. During recovery there was retention of potassium and loss of the excess sodium and chloride. The results of this study were consistent with expectations. Suffice it to say that the metabolic changes in pneumonia are similar to those induced by the administration of ACTH or cortisone. There are not sufficient data to delineate the role of adrenal cortical hyperactivity in accounting for the changes seen.

During the studies on the antipyretic action of ACTH, the opportunity presented itself to observe the effects of this hormone in therapeutic benign tertian malaria in a young paretic. The periodicity of the paroxysms and the height to which the fever rose were not affected by ACTH, but defervescence was slightly accelerated. When the parasites in the blood stream were counted, they were found to be unusually numerous. Two additional patients with induced malaria due to *P. vivax* were therefore given ACTH, and the degree of parasitemia was compared with that in seven control patients. It was apparent that the administration of ACTH was associated with increased numbers of parasites in the blood (20). The studies were extended to the malignant quotidian infection of rhesus monkeys (*Macaca mulatta*) caused by *P. knowlesi* (7, 21). It was found that each of four ACTH-treated monkeys developed hemoglobinuria, whereas only 20 percent of a large control series developed this complication under the standard conditions of the experiment. There is less than one chance in a hundred that the difference in the incidence of hemoglobinuria was the result of chance alone. The survival time of the treated monkeys was no greater than in controls, but the treated monkeys, up to the time of death, showed normal activity and none of the clinical manifestations of acute malaria caused by *P. knowlesi*.

Rodent malaria caused by *P. berghei* is an infection which usually undergoes spontaneous remission. However, when rats were treated with cortisone and infected with this plasmodium, the animals almost always succumbed. In control rats in which spontaneous remission had occurred, the administration of cortisone, if begun within a few days, was usually followed by relapse and death of the host (7). Comparable findings have recently been reported with *P. relictum* in pigeons (22). In this disease, cortisone also induced relapse soon after an attack, but, as in rodent malaria, the relapse could not be induced if remission was prolonged. It has also been shown recently that in benign primate (*M. mulatta*) malaria caused by *P. cynomolgi* parasitemia was greater in treated animals than in controls, and the hormone induced recrudescences in chronically infected monkeys (23).

The observations on malaria were of particular interest, because in this disease the characteristic pathologic changes are not those of acute inflammation. Furthermore, since the predominant defensive mechanism in malaria is the reticulo-endothelial system, these observations suggest that ACTH and cortisone may have inhibited reticulo-endothelial activity.

Further evidence that functional derangement of the reticulo-endothelial system may be induced by cortisone derives from the following observations (7). When a rabbit's own erythrocytes are washed and injected into the rear foot pad, the popliteal node draining the area becomes hyperemic, edematous, and is colored a deep red by the injected erythrocytes, which are seen on section to be largely within the macrophages of the node. Within a day or two, erythrocytes are no longer discernible as such within the macrophages, and within two or three days the red color of erythrocytes has virtually disappeared from the node. In animals treated with cortisone, however, the erythrocytes persisted in the nodes for as long as ten to fourteen days. This observation suggests that, apart from a possible effect on phagocytosis that has been observed by others (24), cortisone may reduce the functional capacity of macrophages to dispose of ingested particles, and the studies reported by Thomas and by Lurie in this symposium are consistent with such an interpretation.

It is also conceivable that cortisone may delay the rate of absorption of injected material from the local site of deposition and hence account for the continued appearance of injected material in the regional nodes of cortisone-treated animals. It is possible that both delayed resorption from the local site and delayed disposition by the phagocytes may result from the injection of cortisone.

The present status of the mechanisms by which ACTH and cortisone may reduce susceptibility to infection is summarized below. These mechanisms have all been discussed in detail at this symposium.

EFFECTS OF ACTH AND CORTISONE WHICH MAY INCREASE
SUSCEPTIBILITY TO INFECTION

1. Inhibition of inflammation
    a. Inhibition of phagocytosis
    b. Decrease of capillary permeability
    c. Decrease of fibrogenesis
2. Inhibition of formation of antibodies
3. Negative nitrogen balance
4. Inhibition of reticulo-endothelial activity

Induced depression of resistance may be of diagnostic aid. It has been shown, for example, that adult mice, usually insusceptible to the Coxsackie viruses, may be rendered susceptible to one of these viruses by pretreatment with cortisone (25–26). This phenomenon has been shown for other viruses as well (26–27). We have attempted to use cortisone as an aid to the establishment of influenza viral infections in mice. Throat washings known to contain virus from studies in eggs were passed through cortisone-treated, as well as control, mice. There were no more frequent recoveries of virus from the hormone-treated animals than from the control animals. Throat washings which were negative in eggs were also invariably negative in cortisone-treated mice. When infected allantoic fluids were passed through mice, animals which had been treated with cortisone frequently succumbed to such viruses with characteristic pulmonary lesions, but serial passage of allantoic fluid virus through cortisone-treated mice did not make the viruses more virulent for control mice (7).

The difference in the effects of ACTH and of cortisone on resistance to infection in experimental animals was previously mentioned. It is not at all clear that this difference exists in man, and there is not, at present, any acceptable evidence that in man one of these hormones is more likely than the other to depress mechanisms of resistance to infection. The differences observed in experimental animals may be explained in several ways.

In the first place, ACTH has usually been given to animals by intraperitoneal or subcutaneous routes. It is now known that these are relatively wasteful routes of injection and that hence only a small proportion of the injected hormone is actually providing a sustained stimulus to endogenous secretion by the adrenal cortices of the host. Furthermore, when sufficiently large doses of cortisone are injected subcutaneously or intramuscularly, the effects of the hormone may be demonstrated for seven to ten days after the last dose. On the other hand, even with large doses of ACTH an effect is rarely sustained for more than twelve hours after intraperitoneal, subcutaneous, or intramuscular injection (7).

Another possible explanation of the difference in the effects of ACTH and cortisone in infections may be that this reflects some species differences in the nature and amount of the adrenal cortical secretions. Only cortisone and hydrocortisone of the steroids so far tested have altered significantly the clinical course of rheumatoid arthritis and related disorders (28). The studies of adrenal vein blood and adrenal gland perfusates indicate that the principal secretions of the adrenal cortex are corticosterone (compound B) and 17-hydroxycorticosterone (compound F, or hydrocortisone). This is true of the glands of oxen and dogs, and there is evidence to suggest that it is also true in man (29–31). However, the ingenious studies with perfused bovine adrenal glands show that although these glands produce relatively large amounts of compounds B and F after initial stimulation with ACTH, repeated stimulation leads to increasing proportions of compound F. If compound B should prove to have no depressant effect on mechanisms of resistance to infection just as it has no anti-arthritic effect, then the effect of ACTH would depend upon the relative amounts of compounds B and F produced by stimulation of the adrenal cortices. It is even conceivable that in some animals steroids other than cortisone or hydrocortisone may be secreted under the influence of ACTH. Such a possibility is supported by the striking finding of Bush (32) that some laboratory animals do not have significant amounts of hydrocortisone in their adrenal glands, but instead appear to make only corticosterone (compound B). These are obviously paths for future investigation.

It has been assumed that the capacity of cortisone and hydrocortisone to reduce inflammation and depress resistance to infection is directly related to the clinical responses induced by these steroids. If this is so, it should follow that compound B, although a product of the adrenal cortex, should have no effect on inflammation or on resistance to infection. This hypothesis is under examination at the present time.

It is also possible that cortisone depresses resistance to infection more than does compound F and that the assumption that depression of resistance is directly related to therapeutic efficacy is incorrect. Such a possibility cannot be dimissed at present, because of the frequency with which investigators have noted that in patients who manifested striking clinical improvement after the administration of ACTH or cortisone there was not always a noticeable decrease in the inflammatory response or in the rate of healing of various lesions. Furthermore, clinical improvement has not necessarily been associated with a decreased capacity of the patient to respond to inflammatory irritants, whether antigenic or nonantigenic, and antibody levels have not always been depressed by ACTH or cortisone. Although these observations may represent only differences of degree, the possibility cannot be excluded that clinical effects and depression of some aspects of resistance may be separable phenomena.

The relative effects of compounds E and F on infection are therefore under investigation. When the acetates of cortisone and hydrocortisone were compared, compound F did not significantly alter resistance, whereas the same amount of cortisone markedly depressed resistance of partially protected mice to pneumococci and to influenza A virus (7). These data are as yet incomplete and may not be pertinent, because it has been shown that compound F acetate is not very active metabolically after intramuscular injection (33), whereas the unesterified material is active by this route. In our experiments the hydrocortisone acetate was given subcutaneously and might not have been effective by this route. Furthermore, it must be shown that in mice the rates of absorption of compounds E and F after subcutaneous administration are comparable if comparisons of activity between the two are to be entirely valid.

It was also of interest to determine whether growth hormone might reverse the effects of cortisone on resistance to infection. Through the kindness of Drs. M. S. Raben and E. B. Astwood we obtained growth hormone of such high potency that 2.5 mg contained between 50 and 100 times as much hormone as was necessary to maintain normal growth in hypophysectomized rats. This amount of growth hormone was given daily to mice and failed to reverse the effect of cortisone on pneumococcal and influenza viral infections (7). This finding is in disagreement with those of other workers and requires further study (34).

A few limited observations that may have some bearing on the mechanism of resistance to infection may be added. It is now recognized that one effect of the administration of ACTH or cortisone is lymphocytopenia, with accompanying evidence in lymphoid structures of lysis of lymphocytes and atrophy of lymph nodes. Furthermore, when antigenic substances are injected into the paws of rabbits, the regional nodes become hyperplastic and there are significant increases in the pentose nucleic acid (PNA) concentrations which coincide with the appearance of antibody in the nodes (35–36). Because cortisone may depress antibody formation in rabbits (37–38) it was of interest to determine the effect of cortisone on the nucleic acid contents of the popliteal lymph nodes of rabbits.

It was found that despite the destruction of lymphocytes and the atrophy of the lymph nodes in the cortisone-treated rabbits, the concentration of desoxyribonucleic acid (DNA) did not change, whereas the concentration of PNA was diminished significantly (39). It appeared that this may explain the depression of antibody formation following the administration of cortisone, for if PNA is necessary for antibody production and its metabolism is altered by the hormones, it is conceivable that synthesis of antibody would be affected. This possibility is under investigation, and preliminary data suggest that the increase in PNA which follows the injection of antigens is significantly less in cortisone-treated rabbits than in untreated controls. These changes in nucleic acid concentration may simply reflect alterations in cellular growth patterns rather than direct interference with PNA metabolism, but they are, nevertheless, of some interest.

From the clinical point of view, the question arises whether there are instances in which ACTH or cortisone should be used solely for their apparently beneficial symptomatic effects. The simultaneous use of antibiotics and of cortisone has been suggested by some workers as a means of abbreviating the acute toxic phase of an infection thereby, perhaps, also shortening the period of convalescence (40–43). This is an interesting line for investigation, but requires great care in order to evaluate it properly. Just as the protective effect of antipneumococcal serum was reduced by cortisone therapy, so it was found that the amount of penicillin which protected mice infected with pneumococci was inadequate to protect similar cortisone-treated mice (7). Some of the observations reported by Thomas at this symposium also indicate a diminished effectiveness of penicillin in cortisone-treated animals.

In experimental tuberculosis the combination of streptomycin and cortisone is less effective than streptomycin alone (44). Finally, it should be pointed out again that in the mice with influenza viral infections cortisone seemed in some manner to reduce the capacity of the host to survive an otherwise nonfatal concentration of virus. Obviously then, great care and proper statistical evaluation of the results will be necessary before it can be decided whether combined cortisone and antimicrobial treatment will prove of value.

Another instance in which the use of ACTH or cortisone may be contemplated is in the treatment of acute adrenal insufficiency that is alleged to occur during infection. This is a most difficult subject to evaluate at present. Such conditions as Waterhouse-Friderichsen syndrome and acute diphtheritic intoxication have become so uncommon that the data on the use of adrenocortical hormones consist of isolated reports that cannot be evaluated against the natural history of these diseases, particularly as they are influenced by modern antimicrobial therapy. In experimental intoxications with diphtherial or meningococcal toxins (45), as in the toxemias induced by the acute toxic action of influenza viruses, rickettsiae, or typhoidal endotoxin, ACTH and cortisone did not lead to increased survival. It is interesting, furthermore, that hemorrhagic adrenal glands resembling some of those seen in the Waterhouse-Friderichsen syndrome were produced in rats not by inducing adrenal insufficiency, but by administering large intravenous doses of ACTH; the hemorrhagic adrenal cortices in this instance were caused by extreme hyperactivity of the glands (46). Finally, it is surprising that despite the relative frequency with which severe diphtherial and meningococcal infections have been observed within the past fifty years, there are, so far as we know, no reports of Addison's disease as a sequel to these infections in patients in whom recovery has been reported. Although many explanations might be advanced for the absence of such cases, it is, nevertheless, noteworthy.

Although the clinical appearance of the patient with vasomotor collapse due to sepsis is consistent with findings in adrenal insufficiency, and pathologic evidence is incontrovertible that damage to the adrenal cortices may occur, it is not yet clear to what extent this damage is specific for the adrenal cortex and not merely a reflection of severe damage to metabolic processes throughout the body. It is even less clear that when toxic bacterial products interfere with cellular metabolism such interference is at that level of cellular activity at which the adrenal cortical hormones play a catalytic role. The problem is complex and will require carefully controlled investigation.

In conclusion, it is worth re-emphasizing that although the studies made with the use of ACTH and cortisone have increased our understanding of the processes of infection and immunity, the clinical use of these hormones in infectious diseases must still be undertaken with caution.

REFERENCES

1. Finland, M., E. H. Kass, and S. H. Ingbar, Effects of ACTH in primary atypical (viral) pneumonia and in pneumococcal pneumonia (preliminary report), *Proc. 1st Clinical ACTH Conference*, ed. by J. R. Mote, The Blakiston Co., Philadelphia, 1950, pp. 529–535.
2. Kass, E. H., S. H. Ingbar, and M. Finland, Effects of adrenocorticotropic hormone in pneumonia: clinical, bacteriological and serological studies, *Ann. Int. Med.*, 1950, 33:1081.
3. Kass, E. H., S. H. Ingbar, M. M. Lundgren and M. Finland, The effect

of ACTH and cortisone on pneumococcal and influenza viral infections in white mice, *J. Lab. & Clin. Med.*, 1951, 37:780.
4. Loosli, C. G., R. B. Hull, B. S. Berlin, and E. R. Alexander, The influence of ACTH on the course of experimental influenza type A virus infection, *J. Lab. & Clin. Med.*, 1951, 37:464.
5. Kass, E. H., F. A. Neva, and M. Finland, Failure of ACTH to protect against acutely lethal toxins of influenza virus and rickettsiae, *Proc. Soc. Exp. Biol. & Med.*, 1951, 76:560.
6. Jackson, E. B., and J. E. Smadel, The effects of cortisone and ACTH on toxins of rickettsiae and *Salmonella typhosa*, *J. Immunol.*, 1951, 66:621.
7. Unpublished observations.
8. Mote, J. R., ed., *Proc. 2d Clin. ACTH Conf.*, The Blakiston Company, Philadelphia, 1951, 2 vols.
9. Kass, E. H., and M. Finland, Effect of ACTH on induced fever, *New England J. Med.*, 1950, 243:693.
10. Duffy, B. J., Jr., and H. R. Morgan, ACTH and cortisone aggravation or suppression of the febrile response of rabbits to bacterial endotoxin, *Proc. Soc. Exp. Biol. & Med.*, 1951, 78:687.
11. Douglas, W. W., and W. D. M. Paton, The hypothermic and antipyretic effect of preparations of ACTH, *Lancet*, 1952, 1:342.
12. Recant, L., Ott, W. H., and E. E. Fischel, The antipyretic effect of cortisone, *Proc. Soc. Exp. Biol. & Med.*, 1950, 75:264.
13. Michael, M., The effect of cortisone and ACTH on bacterial infections, *South. M.J.*, 1951, 44:450.
14. Beck, J. C., J. S. L. Browne, L. J. Johnson, B. J. Kennedy, and D. W. MacKenzie, Occurrence of peritonitis during ACTH administration, *Canad. M.A.J.*, 1950, 62:423.
15. Irons, E., J. Ayer, R. Brown, and S. Armstrong, ACTH and cortisone in diffuse collagen disease and chronic dermatoses; differential therapeutic effects. *J.A.M.A.*, 1951, 145:861.
16. Brunsting, L. A., C. H. Slocumb, and J. W. Didcoct, Effects of cortisone on acute disseminated lupus erythematosus. *Arch. Derm. & Syph.*, 1951, 63:29.
17. Ebert, R. H., Personal communication.
18. Mogabgab, W. J., and L. Thomas, The effects of cortisone on bacterial infections, *J. Lab. & Clin. Med.*, 1952, 39:271.
19. Shwartzman, G., Poliomyelitis infection in cortisone-treated hamsters induced by the intraperitoneal route, *Proc. Soc. Exp. Biol. & Med.*, 1952, 79:573.
20. Kass, E. H., Q. M. Geiman, and M. Finland, Effects of ACTH on induced malaria in man, *New England J. Med.*, 1951, 245:1000.
21. Kass, E. H., Q. M. Geiman, S. H. Ingbar, A. B. Ley, J. W. Harris, and M. Finland, Some diseases which may be activated by ACTH—observations in sickle-cell anemia and malaria, *Proc. 2d Clin. ACTH Conf.*, J. R. Mote, ed., The Blakiston Co., Philadelphia, 1951, II, 376–380.

22. Redmond, W. B., Influence of cortisone on natural course of malaria in the pigeon, *Proc. Soc. Exp. Biol. & Med.*, 1952, 79:258.
23. Schmidt, L. H., and W. L. Squires, The influence of cortisone on primate malaria, *J. Exp. Med.*, 1951, 94:501.
24. Crepea, S. B., G. E. Magnin, and C. V. Seastone, Effect of ACTH and cortisone on phagocytosis, *Proc. Soc. Exp. Biol. & Med.*, 1951, 77:704.
25. Kilbourne, E. D., and F. L. Horsfall, Jr., Lethal infection with Coxsackie virus of adult mice given cortisone, *Proc. Soc. Exp. Biol. & Med.*, 1951, 77:135.
26. Findlay, G. M., and E. M. Howard, The effects of cortisone and adrenocorticotrophic hormone on poliomyelitis and on other virus infection, *J. Pharmacy & Pharmacol.*, 1952, 4:37.
27. Shwartzman, G., Enhancing effect of cortisone upon poliomyelitis infection (strain MEF_1) in hamsters and mice, *Proc. Soc. Exp. Biol. & Med.*, 1950, 75:835.
28. Kendall, E. C., Relation of chemical structure of adrenal cortical hormones to biological activity, in "Adrenal Cortex: Transactions of First Conference," Elaine P. Ralli, ed., Josiah Macy, Jr., Foundation, New York, 1950.
29. Pincus, G., O. Hechter, and A. Zaffaroni, The effect of ACTH upon steroidogenesis by the isolated perfused adrenal gland, in *Proc. 2d Clin. ACTH Conf.*, J. R. Mote, ed., The Blakiston Co., Philadelphia, 1951, I:40–47.
30. Hechter, O., and others, "The nature and the biogenesis of the adrenal secretory product," in Recent Progress in Hormone Research, G. Pincus, ed., Academic Press, New York, 1951, 6:215.
31. Nelson, D. H., L. T. Samuels, and H. Reich, The cortical steroids in mammalian blood after ACTH stimulation, in *Proc. 2d Clin. ACTH Conf.*, J. R. Mote, ed., The Blakiston Co., Philadelphia, 1951, I:49–53.
32. Bush, I. E., Paper chromatographic study of the secretion of the adrenal cortex in various mammalian species, *J. Physiol.*, 1951, 115:12P (Proc. Physiol. Soc. 19 May, 1951).
33. Conn, J. W., L. H. Louis, and S. S. Fajans, The probability that compound F (17-hydroxycorticosterone) is the hormone produced by the normal human adrenal cortex, *Science*, 1951, 113:713.
34. Selye, H., The influence of STH, ACTH and cortisone upon resistance to infection, *Canad. M.A.J.*, 1951, 64:489.
35. Ehrich, W. E., D. L. Drabkin, and C. Forman, Nucleic acids and the production of antibodies by plasma cells, *J. Exp. Med.*, 1949, 90:157.
36. Harris, T. H., and S. Harris, Histochemical changes in lymphocytes during the production of antibodies in lymph nodes of rabbits, *J. Exp. Med.*, 1949, 90:169.
37. Germuth, F. G., Jr., and B. Ottinger, Effect of 17-hydroxy-11-dehydrocorticosterone (Compound E) and ACTH on Arthus reaction and antibody formation in rabbits, *Proc. Soc. Exp. Biol. & Med.*, 1950, 74:815.

38. Bjørneboe, M., E. E. Fischel, and H. C. Stoerk, The effect of cortisone and adrenocorticotrophic hormone on the concentration of circulating antibody, *J. Exp. Med.*, 1951, 93:37.
39. Kass, E. H., and M. I. Kendrick, Effect of cortisone on nucleoproteins of lymph nodes, *Fed. Proc.*, 1952, 2:472.
40. Kinsell, L. W., The clinical application of pituitary adrenocorticotropic and adrenal steroid hormones, *Ann. Int. Med.*, 1951, 35:615.
41. Hurtig, A., Use of cortisone and antibiotics in resistant pelvic infections, *Postgrad. Med.*, 1952, 2:196.
42. Smadel, J. E., H. L. Ley, and F. H. Diercks, Treatment of typhoid fever; I: Combined therapy with cortisone and chloramphenicol, *Ann. Int. Med.*, 1951, 34:1.
43. Woodward, J. E., H. E. Hall, R. Dias-Rivera, J. E. Hightower, E. Martinez, and R. T. Parker, Treatment of typhoid fever; II: Control of clinical manifestations with cortisone, *Ann. Int. Med.*, 1951, 34:10.
44. Spain, D. W., and N. Molomut, Effects of cortisone in the development of tuberculous lesions in guinea pigs and on their modification by streptomycin therapy, *Am. Rev. Tuberc.*, 1950, 62:337.
45. Murray, R., and S. Branham, Effect of cortisone and ACTH on adrenals in experimental diphtheria, Shiga and meningococcus intoxication, *Proc. Soc. Exp. Biol. & Med.*, 1951, 78:750.
46. Ingle, D. J., The functional interrelationship of the anterior pituitary and the adrenal cortex, *Ann. Int. Med.*, 1951, 35:652.

Chapter 14

ALTERATION OF EXPERIMENTAL POLIOMYELITIS BY MEANS OF CORTISONE WITH REFERENCE TO OTHER VIRUSES [1]

By GREGORY SHWARTZMAN AND STANLEY M. ARONSON, *The Department of Microbiology, The Mount Sinai Hospital, New York, N.Y.*

SOME PREVIOUS EXPERIMENTS have already suggested a relationship between endocrine imbalance and predisposition to poliomyelitis. Thus, Curley and Aycock (1) reported some years ago that castration induced in monkeys a greater susceptibility to the intranasal inoculation of the virus, while the treatment of the castrates with estrogen increased their resistance.

In approaching this problem the relatively higher incidence of poliomyelitis in pregnant women was of particular interest. Since it was clearly shown by Venning (2) that there is a greatly enhanced adrenocortical function during pregnancy, a study on the effect of cortisone on experimental poliomyelitis was suggested. In view of the fact that an enhanced susceptibility rather than protection against the infection was expected, a partially refractory animal was selected for these studies. In connection with other previous studies we became familiar with the behavior of the virus in the Syrian golden hamster. Intracerebral inoculation of a rodent-pathogenic strain of the virus (Lansing or MEF_1) into this animal gives rise to a mild disease of irregular onset, low incidence, and low mortality rate. As judged from observations on hundreds of hamsters, virus diluted 1:20 gives some 50 percent paralysis with an incubation period varying from four to nineteen days. The mortality rate varies from 20 to 40 percent, the mean mortality rate being a little more than 24 percent.

In preliminary experiments the administration of large doses of cortisone alone or ACTH and cortisone in combination induced a prompt and violent infection. Within a day or two after inoculation the treated hamsters appeared weak and drowsy. They showed swollen eyelids, conjunctivitis, ruffled fur, and hunched backs. The paralysis occurred

[1] Aided by a grant from the National Foundation for Infantile Paralysis, Inc.

as early as one to three days following inoculation and was extensive, involving all extremities of some animals, while the control animals rarely showed tetraplegia. The disease was uniformly fatal. In extending the initial observations, it seemed first necessary to find the minimal amount of cortisone required for the enhancement of poliomyelitis infection and to determine the minimal amount of virus capable of eliciting the disease in cortisone treated hamsters.

Comparison of experimental groups receiving doses of 5 mg of cortisone and less and virus diluted 1:20, the controls receiving the same amount of virus, served to determine the minimal amount of cortisone necessary for the enhancement. Since the mean mortality rate in a large group of controls under observation concurrently was 24.6, it is obvious that a mortality rate ranging from 77.8 to 100 percent demonstrates a clear-cut enhancement of the infection with the aid of cortisone. Thus, a single injection of 2 mg of cortisone is sufficient to produce an unequivocal enhancement of the infection. The effect of 1 mg of cortisone giving rise to 55 percent mortality may be considered as the end-point. Single injections of 2 and 5 mg of cortisone given simultaneously with the virus two and eighteen hours prior to virus and eighteen hours after virus are capable of producing approximately the same increase in mortality rate. In contrast, while 5 mg of cortisone are capable of raising the mortality rate to 77.8 percent when injected as long as forty-eight hours prior to virus, a dose of 2 mg fails to do so. In the remaining experiments dealing with virus diluted 1:1000 a mortality rate of 33 to 55 percent was obtained, as against no mortality in the controls.

In addition to increasing the mortality rate, cortisone is also responsible for shortening the mean survival time, death occurring within considerably fewer days than in the control group. A statistical analysis of some of the data using the Student's t-test, kindly carried out by Dr. Franklin Hollander, is given in Table 1.

The administration of cortisone invariably produces a change in the clinical course in the hamster. Several days after inoculation the animals show conjunctivitis, ruffled fur, and arched backs. Neurological symptoms are marked, and tetraplegias are seen much more frequently than in the controls. The incubation period for the onset of paralysis is decidedly shortened, ranging in most animals from three to six days, the highest incidence of paralysis occurring from four to five days following inoculation.

TABLE 1

STATISTICAL ANALYSIS OF ENHANCEMENT OF POLIOMYELITIS INFECTION IN HAMSTERS WITH THE AID OF CORTISONE

HAMSTERS INOCULATED INTERCEREBRALLY WITH MEF_1 DILUTED 1:20

	Controls receiving no cortisone, inoculated with the virus simultaneously with the experimental groups	Cortisone 5 mg 1 × 2 hrs. prior to virus inoculation	Cortisone 2 mg 1 × 18 hrs. prior to virus inoculation	Cortisone 1 mg 1 × immediately prior to virus inoculation	Cortisone 1 mg 1 × 18 hrs. prior to virus inoculation
N	18	10	9	9	10
Range of survival time, days	4–25	3–8	3–11	6–20	7–11
Mean survival time, days	13.8	6.3	5.6	9.8	8.3
P value		0.0008 [a]	0.0007 [a]	0.19 [b]	0.14 [b]

From *J. Exp. Med.*, 1952, 95:347.
[a] Highly significant. [b] Doubtful significance.

TABLE 2

EFFECT OF CORTISONE UPON THE TITER OF MEF_1 IN THE BRAIN OF THE HAMSTER

VIRUS (MEF_1) USED FOR TITRATION	LD_{50} TITER	
	In mice	In hamsters
Pool I		
Stock mouse brain passage	$10^{-3.34}$	$10^{-1.55}$
Pool II		
Brains of 4 hamsters infected with pool I	$10^{-1.63}$	$10^{-2.05}$
Pool III		
Brains of 3 cortisone-treated hamsters infected with pool I	$10^{-3.66}$	$10^{-3.34}$
Pool IV		
Brains of 4 cortisone-treated hamsters infected with pool I	$10^{-3.76}$	n.d.[a]
Pool V		
Brains of hamsters infected with pool III	$10^{-1.27}$	$10^{-1.44}$

From *J. Exp. Med.*, 1952, 95:347.
[a] n.d. = Not determined.

Thus, it may be concluded from a long series of experiments that cortisone produces a highly significant enhancement of experimental poliomyelitis infection in the hamster which results in shortening the incubation period for the onset of paralysis, greater severity of symptoms, marked reduction in the mean survival time, and an increase in the mortality rate to 100 percent. This alteration of the disease is also accompanied by an increased rate of multiplication of the virus under the influence of cortisone (3–4). The observations reported have been amply corroborated by Sabin (5) and Findlay and Howard (6).

When considered in the light of the effect of cortisone just described, a number of previous observations, seemingly unrelated, dealing with the alteration of predisposition to clinical and experimental poliomyelitis may have one common denominator—a possible temporary disturbance in the adrenocortical function and a resulting hypersecretion of cortisone. Therefore they merit reexamination with regard to increased susceptibility due to excessive fatigue in monkeys (7) and man (8–9), surgical procedures and trauma in man and monkeys (10–14), pregnancy in women (15–17) and mice (18–19), prophylactic vaccination in man (20–25), and injection of T.A.B. and pertussis vaccines and diphtheria toxoid in mice (26–27). The effect of cortisone is altogether different from that of other hormones, including ACTH.

The findings that ACTH fails to modify the experimental infection are consistent with the observations of Coriell, Cook, Murphy, and Stokes (28) on the lack of effect of the hormone upon clinical poliomyelitis. However, according to Ainslie, Francis, and Brown (29) and Foster, Sigel, Henle, and Stokes (30) there may be some shortening of the incubation period and a somewhat higher incidence of paralysis in monkeys following the administration of ACTH. The important physiological basis for the possible difference between ACTH and cortisone was pointed out in the introductory remarks opening this symposium. The observations mentioned suggest that further study is needed in order to determine whether ACTH stimulates the elaboration, by the adrenal cortex, of factors other than cortisone which may be opposing the enhancing effect of cortisone.

In extending the observations on the enhancement of the infection by means of cortisone it was deemed of particular interest to determine what effect the cortisone may have on the route of invasion of the

TABLE 3

EFFECT OF VARIOUS HORMONES UPON POLIOMYELITIS IN HAMSTERS

GROUP NO.	TREATMENT	MEF₁ STOCK MOUSE PASSAGE		TOTAL NO. ANIMALS	NEUROLOGICAL SYMPTOMS Days after inoculation	DEATHS Days after inoculation	MEAN SURVIVAL TIME Days	MORTALITY RATE Percentage
		Dilution	Time inoculated					
1	Cortisone 5 mg 3× 4, 19 hrs.	1:20	2 hrs. after 1st cortisone	10	5,5,5,5,5	5,ᵃ5,ᵃ5,ᵃ 5,ᵃ5,ᵃ6, 6,6,6,7.	5.6	100
2	Cortisone 5 mg 1×	1:20	2 hrs. after cortisone	10	2,2,3,3,3, 3,3,3, 6,6	3,6,6,6,6, 7,7,7,7,8 8	6.3	100
3	ACTH 5 mg 3× 4, 19 hrs.	1:20	2 hrs. after 1st ACTH	9	3,6,6	6,10	8.0	22.2
4	ACTH 3 mg 5× 4, 19, 24, 24 hrs.	1:20	2 hrs. after 1st ACTH	9	4,4,7,9	7,7	7.0	22.2
5	ACTH in gelatin 10 mg 2× 24 hrs.	1:20	2 hrs. after 1st ACTH	10	3,5,6,8,14	6,26	16.0	20
6	DCA 1 mg 1×	1:20	½ hr. after DCA	10	8,8			0
7	DCA 1 mg 3× 18, 4 hrs.	1:20	22 hrs. after 3d DCA	8	5,9,11,12	11,15,16, 20	15.5	50

GROUP NO.	TREATMENT	MEF₁ STOCK MOUSE PASSAGE		TOTAL NO. ANIMALS	NEUROLOGICAL SYMPTOMS Days after inoculation	DEATHS Days after inoculation	MEAN SURVIVAL TIME Days	MORTALITY RATE Percentage
		Dilution	Time inoculated					
8	DCA 1 mg 3× 18, 4, 18 hrs. Cortisone 5 mg 3× 4, 18 hrs.	1:20	2 hrs. after 1st cortisone	10	1,1,1,1,1, 1,5,5	1,[a]2,2,5,5, 5,[a]6,6,7, 7	5.8	100
9	Progesterone 0.25 mg 3× 24, 24 hrs.	1:20	Immediately after 2d progesterone	10	5,14,22	25	25.0	10
10	Diethylstilbestrol 0.25 mg 3× 24, 24 hrs.	1:20	Immediately after 2d stilbestrol	10	4,4,7	19,19	19.0	20
Controls for 1–10	No treatment	1:20	...	50	3,4,4,4,5, 5,6,6,6, 6,6,7,7, 7,7,7,7, 8,8,9,9, 9,12,14, 19,19	4,[a]5,6,7, 9,9,10, 14,19	8.3	18
11	ACTH 5 mg 1× Cortisone 5 mg 2× 5, 19 hrs.	1:100	3 hrs. after ACTH	10	2,2,2,2,3, 3,3,3,3, 3	4,6,6,6,6, 6,6,7,9, 10	6.6	100
Control for 11	No treatment	1:100	...	10	6,6,6,7,9, 20	15,21	18.0	20

From *J. Exp. Med.*, 1952, 95:347.
[a] Died without neurological symptoms.

virus. The Lansing strain of poliomyelitis virus invades the rodent only by the intracerebral route. Following the intraperitoneal injection of massive doses there is a rapid disappearance of the virus, no trace of it being recovered in any organ a few hours later. In our experiments, hamsters received several intramuscular injections of cortisone and an intraperitoneal inoculation of the virus strain MEF_1. A severe disease was thus elicited.

TABLE 4

MEF_1 INFECTION IN HAMSTERS BY THE INTRAPERITONEAL ROUTE

Total Number	Treatment with Cortisone	Time of Inoculation	Inoculum Dilution	Paralysis Onset Range of Days	Mean Survival Time	Mortality Rate, %
121	...	...	1:20 to 1:12000	...	...	0
45	2 mg 4× 24, 27, 20 hr.	...	...	...	14.0	6.0
10	2 mg 1×	2 hr. after cortisone	1:20	5–6	7.3	30
10	5 mg 1×	Immed. after cortisone	1:20	6–16	12	60
10	2 mg 2× 24 hr.	2 hr. after 2d cortisone	1:20	5–8	7.4	100
10	2 mg 3× 19, 27 hr.	Immed. after 3d cortisone	1:1000	4–10	8	66.7
10	2 mg 4× 24, 27, 20 hr.	Immed. after 3d cortisone	1:100	3–5	4.7	100
15		Immed. after 3d cortisone	1:500	5–10	8	100
10		Immed. after 3d cortisone	1:1000	5–9	7.6	55.5
10		Immed. after 3d cortisone	1:8000	5–12	9	60
10		Immed. after 3d cortisone	1:12000	4–11	...	0
10	3 mg 3× 19, 24 hr.	2½ hr. after 3d cortisone	1:20	4–7	6.5	100
10	3 mg 4× 4, 20, 3 hr.	Immed. after 3d cortisone	1:100	3–5	5.5	100.0

From *Proc. Soc. Exp. Biol. & Med.*, 1952, 79:573.

There is ample proof that the disease elicited in this manner is true experimental poliomyelitis.

1. There was obtained a typical clinical disease in a great majority of animals frequently resulting in tetraplegia. Characteristic histological

changes were invariably seen in the spinal cord in the animals showing the disease during life.

2. The virus recovered from the brain of the intraperitoneally infected hamsters produced typical symptoms in mice, the recovery of the virus coinciding with the development of the disease. The virus was neutralized by the anti-Lansing convalescent monkey serum on intracerebral testing in mice. In these titrations 200 mouse LD_{50} were completely neutralized by the serum diluted 1:10 following incubation of the mixture for one hour in a water bath at 37°C.

3. It was also possible to neutralize the virus in the hamsters. In these experiments the hamsters received four injections of 2 mg of cortisone at intervals of three, twenty, and three hours. One-half ml. of suitable dilutions of virus and serum incubated in a water bath at 37°C for one hour were injected intraperitoneally immediately following the fourth injection of cortisone. There was obtained consistent neutralization of the virus diluted 1:500 with the serum diluted 1:40, while in the absence of the serum the virus similarly diluted and incubated gave 100 percent mortality, with a mean survival time of five days.

A fact of outstanding interest is that the animals showed a marked viremia, the extent of which depended largely on the total dose of cortisone, the frequency of administration, and the concentration of the inoculated virus.

The results indicate an extraneural multiplication of the poliomyelitis virus following the intraperitoneal inoculation into cortisone-treated hamsters.

In a later report a good correlation will be demonstrated between histological changes and the concentration of the virus in certain organs and tissues outside the central nervous system. The results are of special interest in connection with the pathogenesis of the disease, because they suggest that extraneural multiplication of the virus may be one of the phases of the infection following parenteral introduction of the virus. The demonstration by Bodian (31) and Horstmann (32) of a viremia in the chimpanzee following feeding of the virus, points in the same direction.

The possibility of producing the infection by the intraperitoneal route offers a new method for intraperitoneal testing of neutralizing potency of sera and for investigating the effect of chemotherapeutic agents before fixation of the virus by the central nervous system. Other distinct

TABLE 5

RECOVERY OF VIRUS FROM HAMSTERS INFECTED INTRAPERITONEALLY

Treatment with cortisone	MEF$_1$ Inoculum dilution	ORGAN TESTED Name	Hr. after inoculation	Dilution	Result in mice [b]
...	1:20	Brain	96	1:20	0/8
5 mg 1×	1:20		20	1:20	0/7
	1:20		70	1:20	0/8
	1:20		192	1:20	5/8
...	1:20	Serum	96	1:2	0/8
5 mg 1×	1:20		70	1:10	0/6
	1:20		192	1:10	0/6
2 mg 2× 24 hrs.	1:20		23	1:10	1/16
	1:20		23	1:100	0/16
	1:20		96	1:10	13/16
	1:20		96	1:100	2/16
3 mg 3× 19, 24 hrs.	1:20	Brain	96	1:100 [a]	6/6
	1:20	Serum	96	1:10	11/16
	1:20		96	1:100	4/16
3 mg 4× 4, 20, 3 hrs.	1:100	Brain	120	1:100	6/6
	1:100		120	1:1000	5/6
	1:100		120	1:5000 [a]	5/6
	1:100	Serum	120	1:10	6/6
	1:100		120	1:100	2/6
	1:100		120	1:1000	1/6
5 mg 4× 19, 24, 24 hrs.	1:1000		72	1:10	6/6
	1:1000		72	1:100	3/6
	1:1000		72	1:1000	0/6
	1:1000		120	1:10	6/6
	1:1000		120	1:100	6/6
	1:1000		120	1:1000	5/6
	1:1000		120	1:4000	1/6

[a] Higher dilutions not tested.
[b] Numerator = no. of dead animals; denominator = total no. of animals tested.
Source: *Proc. Soc. Exp. Biol. & Med.*, 1952, 79:573.

advantages of this method result from the fact that by adjusting the dosage of cortisone and the concentration of the virus it may be possible to obtain various degrees of severity of the disease, ranging from a prolonged incubation period and low mortality rate to a uniformly severe disease of short incubation period and high mortality rate, thus affording the opportunity to screen agents under widely different conditions.

The fact that the effects described are not limited to a single animal species is brought out by experiments on monkeys. Thus far good evidence is suggested that there is a rather marked increase of takes following the intramuscular inoculation of the Brunhilde strain in the cortisone-treated Rhesus monkeys. Five control monkeys receiving Brunhilde diluted 1:100 intramuscularly showed no evidence of clinical poliomyelitis during the six-week period of observation. In the experimental group there were nine monkeys treated with cortisone and inoculated intramuscularly with Brunhilde diluted 1:100. Seven monkeys developed an extremely severe poliomyelitis infection five to twelve days following inoculation of the virus. An ascending paralysis of Landry type involved all extremities and abdominal and chest muscles. The eighth monkey had limited paralysis, and the ninth monkey died before the onset of paralysis. Furthermore, from our studies and those of Sabin (5), it appears that strains nonparalytic for monkeys can be made to induce a severe prostrating paralysis following treatment with cortisone.

Thus, a general rule becomes obvious. When the virus is of sufficiently high virulence or when a sufficient concentration of virus invades a highly susceptible host, the virus can do the job for itself under normal physiological conditions in the host. However, when the host is partially refractory or the virus is of low virulence for the host, the hormone may enhance the disease extraordinarily by allowing greater multiplication of the virus, by increasing markedly the severity of neurological symptoms, and by allowing the entry of the virus through parenteral ordinarily refractory routes.

Histological studies on hamsters and monkeys similar to the investigations recorded above were undertaken to delineate any morphologic changes which might be correlated with the phenomenon of poliomyelitis enhancement by means of cortisone following intracerebral and intraperitoneal inoculation of strain MEF_1.

A group of two hundred and eighty male hamsters furnished the source for a detailed pathological survey. The animals were divided into appropriate control groups and experimental groups, as described in Table 6; Groups I, II, VI, and VII provided the tissues for comparative studies on the effects of the MEF_1 virus. Information concerning the effects of cortisone upon reactive and reparative intracranial activity, exclusive of the action of the infectious agent, was derived from hamsters in Groups III and IV. Groups VIII and IX afforded data on peritoneal reaction to nonspecific inocula and the effects of cortisone upon this response. A baseline of tissue changes attributable to cortisone alone was derived from Groups V and X.

Animals from all groups were sacrificed at daily intervals. The brains were serially sectioned. Spinal cords and encasing osseous and soft-tissue structures were sectioned at appropriate levels. Sympathetic ganglia were isolated with the help of a dissecting microscope and examined histologically. All visceral organs were sectioned. Hematoxylin and eosin were used routinely. In addition, a wide range of special stains was employed when needed.

Following intracerebral inoculation the host reaction to the intracranial needle tract was considerably modified in animals receiving cortisone (Figs. 1–2). The cellular and vascular responsiveness which characterized the reaction to cerebral injury was significantly delayed and inhibited. In animals receiving no cortisone which were sacrificed on the first day (Table 6, Groups II and IV), prompt leukocyte migration to the needle tract was seen. In cortisone-treated animals sacrificed at the same time (Table 6, Groups I and III), the tissues adjacent to the traumatic tract were totally quiescent. After the fourth day there was a perceptible degree of reparation of the needle tract in the control hamsters. The hemorrhage incident to the intracerebral inoculation was largely resorbed and the numerous activated microglia congregated about the line of injury were distended with hemosiderin inclusions. While inflammatory infiltration, vascular hyperplasia (Fig. 3), and microglial congregation were prominent in animals receiving no cortisone, these changes were absent, subdued, or belatedly present when the hormone was previously administered.

A similar pattern of mesodermal inhibition was recognized in areas of neuronal damage due to the virus. When cortisone was not admin-

TABLE 6

EXPERIMENTAL PROCEDURE

GROUP	Number of Hamsters	Inoculum	Route	Cortisone
I	40	0.05 cc MEF$_1$ stock mouse brain passage diluted 1:20 (LD$_{50}$ = $10^{-3.7}$)	Intracerebral	5 mgm I.M., 1× with intracerebral inoculation
II	40	0.05 cc MEF$_1$ stock mouse brain passage diluted 1:20 (LD$_{50}$ = $10^{-3.7}$)	Intracerebral	None
III	5	0.05 cc sterile mouse brain emulsion diluted 1:20.	Intracerebral	5 mgm I.M., 1× with intracerebral inoculation
IV	5	0.05 cc sterile mouse brain emulsion diluted 1:20.	Intracerebral	None
V	10	None	—	5 mgm I.M., 1× with intracerebral inoculation
VI	40	0.5 cc MEF$_1$ stock mouse brain passage diluted 1:20	Intraperitoneal	3 mgm I.M., 4× day prior to and day of I.P. inoc.
VII	40	0.5 cc MEF$_1$ stock mouse brain passage diluted 1:20	Intraperitoneal	None
VIII	5	0.5 cc sterile mouse brain emulsion diluted 1:20	Intraperitoneal	3 mgm I.M., 4× day prior to and day of I.P. inoc.
IX	5	0.5 cc sterile mouse brain emulsion diluted 1:20	Intraperitoneal	None
X	10	None	—	3 mgm I.M., 4× day prior to and day of I.P. inoc.

istered, the mesenchymal response to viral neuronolysis was prompt and exhuberant (Fig. 4). Leukocytes migrated rapidly to the damaged neurons, and phagocytic elements accumulated around the cells undergoing degeneration. The endothelium of neighboring blood vessels became hyperplastic. The surrounding perivascular spaces were distended, with inflammatory cells. A diffuse meningitis was visible. The necrobiotic aspect of the disease was thus overshadowed by the supervening host response. When cortisone was given at the time of intracerebral inoculation, neuronolysis proceeded in a unilateral fashion, usually unattended by the classical features of neuronophagia, parenchymal infiltration, and perivascular cuffing (Fig. 5). After cell destruction was accomplished, an indolent and impoverished reaction developed. The mitigating action of cortisone upon scavenger activity resulted in the persistence of anuclear fragments of necrotic cytoplasm in the sites previously occupied by neurons.

Generally speaking, the number of neurons destroyed was greater in infected hamsters receiving adjuvant cortisone. The hippocampal cortex affords an excellent site for quantitative comparison. This cerebral region forms a significant portion of the rodent brain, shows a cytoarchitectonic pattern of neurons which is clearly linear and is uniquely susceptible to the action of many rodent-adapted neurotropic viruses. In addition, the intracerebral inoculum is usually deposited within its white matter. In the absence of cortisone administration, hippocampal involvement was sparse, usually restricted to the side corresponding to the needle tract terminus, and marked by florid inflammatory response. Hamsters treated with cortisone, on the other hand, disclosed extensive and often plenary neuronolysis. Many animals surviving beyond the sixth day showed complete hippocampal acellularity, with lines of empty vacuoles sometimes bearing necrotic detritus (Fig. 6). Bilateral involvement was almost constantly observed, often with precise symmetry. Neighboring blood vessels appeared unaffected by the fulminant necrosis.

When the disease was not enhanced by cortisone, the establishment of neuronolytic lesions was never rostral to the inoculum depot and only occasionally contralateral in the cortex. In contrast, cortisone administration allowed both contralateral and rostral involvement and severe olfactory bulb destruction (Figs. 7–8) during the late stages of the

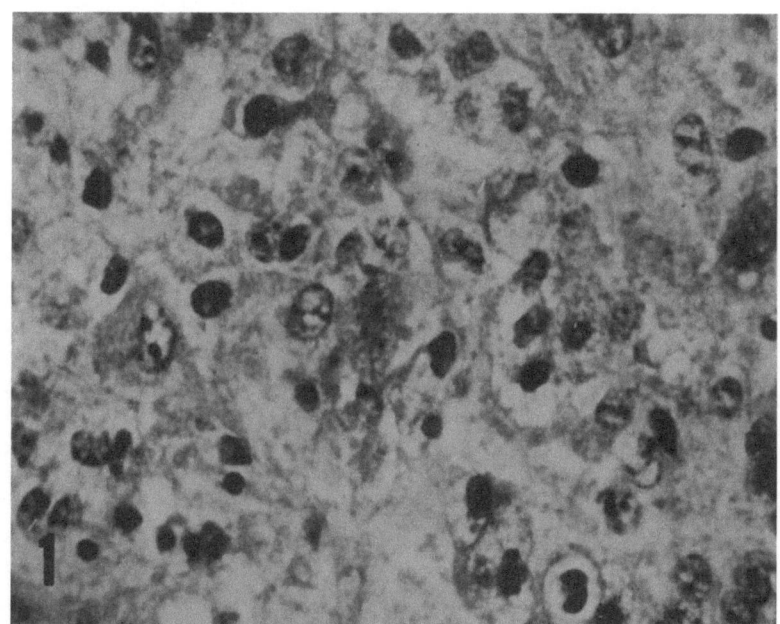

FIGURE 1. NEEDLE TRACT IN HAMSTER INOCULATED INTRACEREBRALLY WITH MEF_1; NO CORTISONE
Sacrificed after four days; traumatic defect filled with reactive cells; hemorrhage resorbed; H & E ×500.

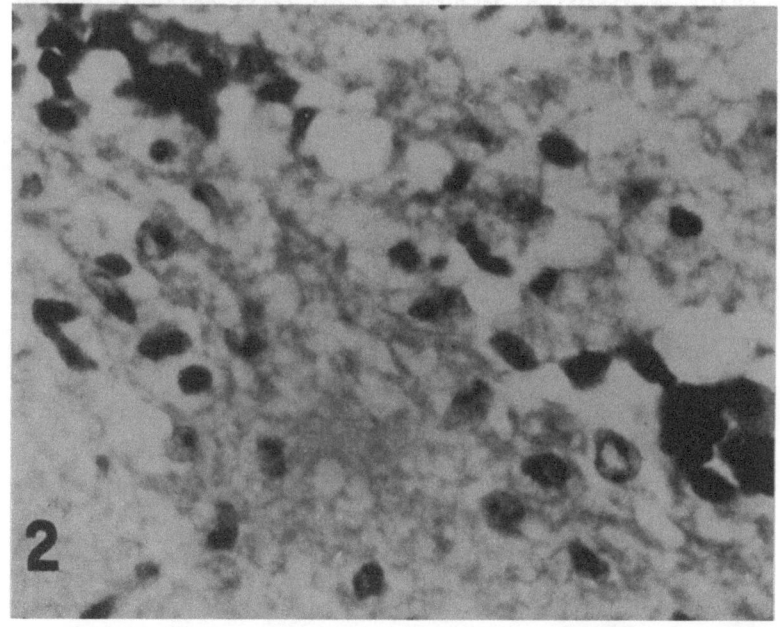

FIGURE 2. NEEDLE TRACT IN HAMSTER INOCULATED INTRACEREBRALLY WITH MEF_1: CORTISONE GIVEN INTRAMUSCULARLY
Sacrificed after four days; minimal response to injury seen; much of the hemorrhage still persistent; H & E ×500.

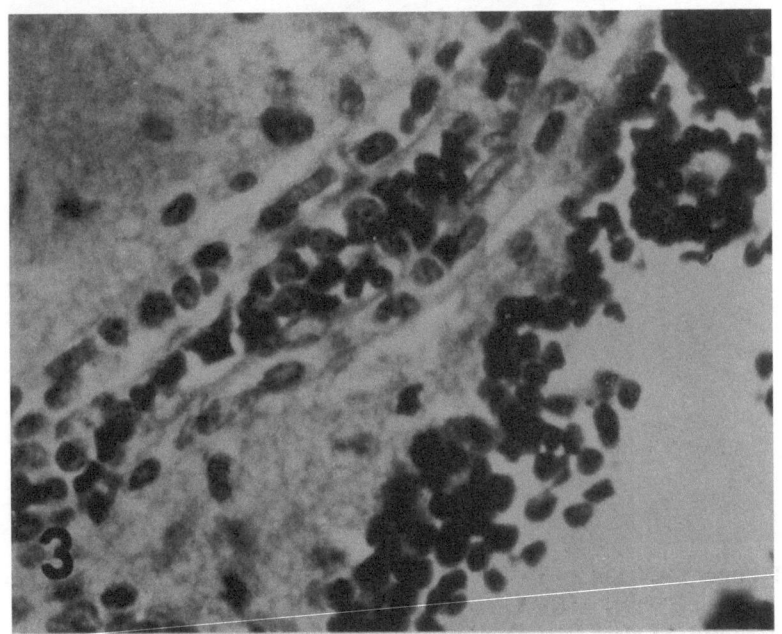

FIGURE 3. PARENCHYMAL BLOOD VESSEL ADJACENT TO NEEDLE TRACT IN HAMSTER SACRIFICED TWO DAYS AFTER INTRACEREBRAL INOCULATION OF MEF_1: NO CORTISONE
Note prominence of endothelial elements; H & E ×500.

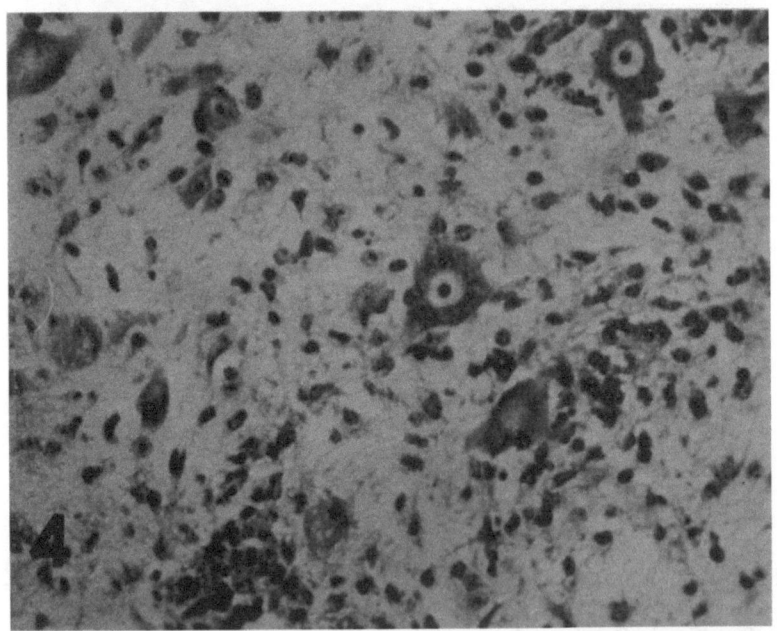

FIGURE 4. POLIOMYELITIS IN THE HAMSTER WITHOUT CORTISONE
Anterior horn showing inflammatory infiltration and prompt neuronophagia; thionine ×250.

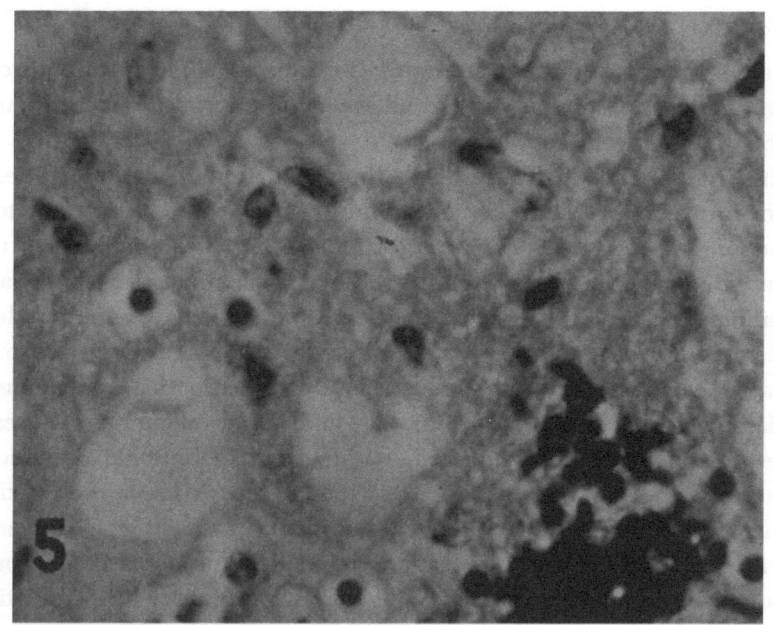

FIGURE 5. POLIOMYELITIS IN THE CORTISONE-TREATED HAMSTER
Anterior horn neurons fallen out and no mesodermal response; H & E ×500.

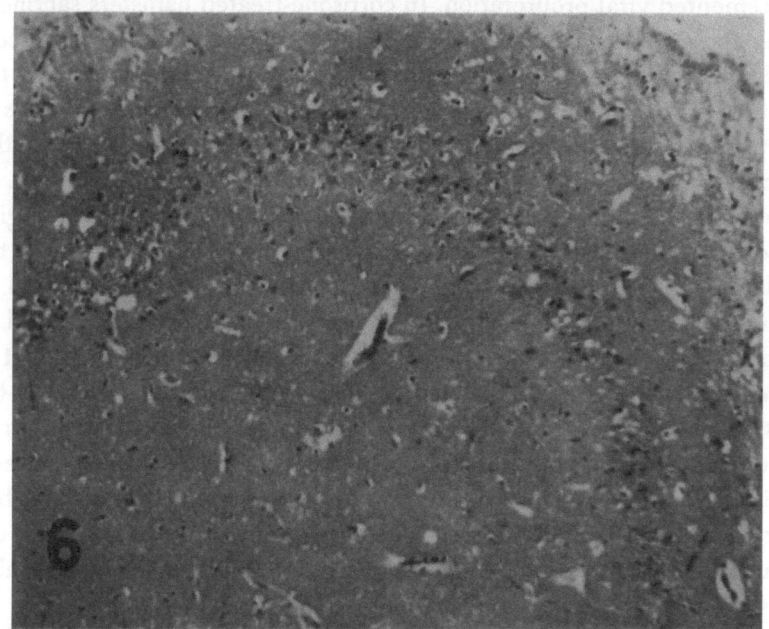

FIGURE 6. HIPPOCAMPAL GYRUS IN CORTISONE-TREATED HAMSTER INFECTED INTRACEREBRALLY WITH MEF$_1$
Massive destruction of neuronal layer with many anuclear remnants; H & E ×100.

disease. Expressed in different terms, it can be concluded that cortisone permits diffusion of the virus to all encephalic zones potentially amenable to viral proliferation.

Inflammation can be considered the summation of all cellular reactions provoked by cell injury. Furthermore, the degree of inflammatory reaction is directly proportional to the degree of this stimulus. In untreated hamsters subjected to intracerebral inoculation of MEF_1 strain, a minimal degree of neurocytolysis evoked an immediate and abundant inflammatory reaction. In the early stages of the disease cortisone-treated hamsters show pronounced neuronal destruction and minimal inflammation. When the necrobiotic (viral) and inflammatory (reactive) components are evaluated, within the experimental conditions described above, it becomes apparent that an inverted reciprocity exists (that is, greater necrobiosis, with diminished inflammation). It cannot be inferred that the restrained response is a result of increased neuronal injury; rather, that the mediating agency which inhibits inflammation also, by other means, allows greater viral proliferation. These two end results of cortisone action are not mutually exclusive, since the limitation of initial cellular defenses is undoubtedly one factor in permitting incremented viral proliferation. In cortisone-treated hamsters sacrificed after the sixth day some central nervous system levels disclose perceptible inflammation, while other levels (in the same animal) display the picture of mesodermal inhibition so characteristic of the initial days of cortisone altered poliomyelitis. In many animals demonstrating this variable picture, an understandable distributional pattern emerges. In the midcerebral areas (the site of inoculation and therefore the region of earliest viral effect) the neuronal destruction is rampant, while the inflammatory aspect is moderate or nonexistent. At levels rostral or caudal to the plane of inoculation the response is more pronounced. It can be demonstrated that the distance from the inoculum depot is directly proportional to the degree of mesodermal reactivity. As the pathogen reaches different central nervous system levels at progressively later periods, the effect of cortisone upon the state of tissue reactivity is mitigated, giving rise to the gradient responsiveness described above. Belated reaction does not occur at sites of earlier neuronal destruction, probably because the products of cell lysis which are capable of stimulating reaction have been effectively dissipated.

The absence of prompt phagocytic response to the necrosis of ganglion cells allows visualization of neuronolysis unimpeded by concomitant scavenger activity. The usual course of early ganglionic degeneration in poliomyelitis consists of chromatolysis, cell distortion, and nuclear eccentricity, pyknosis, or fading. These features are based upon studies in simian poliomyelitis. The disease in hamsters is comparatively more rapid, and early phases of degeneration are rarely seen (Fig. 9). Acidophilic necrosis is most often the initial evidence of ganglionic impairment. The cytoplasm of these cells assumes an intensely eosinophilic granular appearance, followed shortly by cell membrane dissolution and cell fragmentation (Fig. 10). The ragged disintegration of the neuron often occurs with such unseeming haste that a detectable nucleus is still visible in one of the disassociated cell fragments. Hemorrhage into the periganglionic space often occurs at this stage (Fig. 12). Not infrequently only a tissue space indicates the former residence of a neuron (Fig. 5). In the absence of phagocytosis it is difficult to explain the rapid disappearance of the necrotic detritus. Often, and more commonly in the brain than in the spinal cord, a hazy, shrunken, poorly defined anuclear sphere of cytoplasm persists. These cytoplasmic ghosts occasionally contain a few leukocyte inclusions (Fig. 11). In instances of fulminant disease in which death follows closely after the onset of paralysis, changes in the anterior horn neurons may be limited to shrinkage, a questionable criterion of neurocytolysis. Vacuolization of the cytoplasm, still another variant of cellular degeneration, at times is extensive enough to obscure all other features of neuronal degradation. The greater tendency toward acute eosinophilic necrosis cannot be ascribed to any mitigation of intracranial defenses; it must be considered a reflection of the demonstrably heightened viral concentration in the brains of those hamsters receiving cortisone.

As previously mentioned, the intraperitoneal inoculation of the virus into animals receiving concomitant cortisone invariably produced a lethal paralytic disease. When the hormone was omitted none of the animals developed paralysis (although very rarely a hamster disclosed a few subclinical lesions within the spinal cord). The peritoneal cavity contained a sparse exudate, and the mesothelial cells were prominent. Cortisone tended to lessen this response. No local changes attributable to the virus could be demonstrated in either control or experimental groups. The first changes within the central nervous system in cortisone-treated hamsters were seen in the spinal cord, usually the lumbar seg-

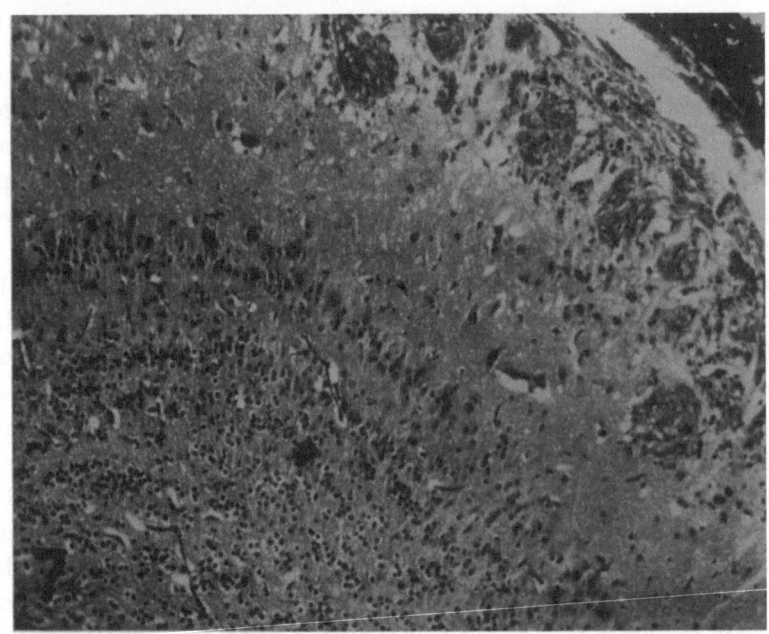

FIGURE 7. OLFACTORY BULB
Normal microscopic appearance; H & E ×250.

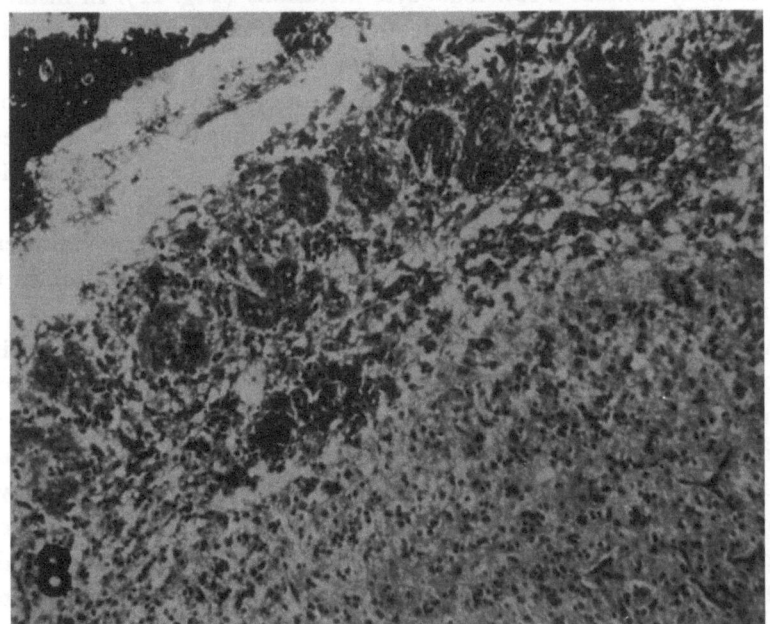

FIGURE 8. OLFACTORY BULB IN CORTISONE-TREATED HAMSTER INOCULATED INTRACEREBRALLY WITH MEF$_1$ AND SACRIFICED EIGHT DAYS LATER
Complete neuronolysis of mitral cell layer and marked inflammatory response; H & E ×250.

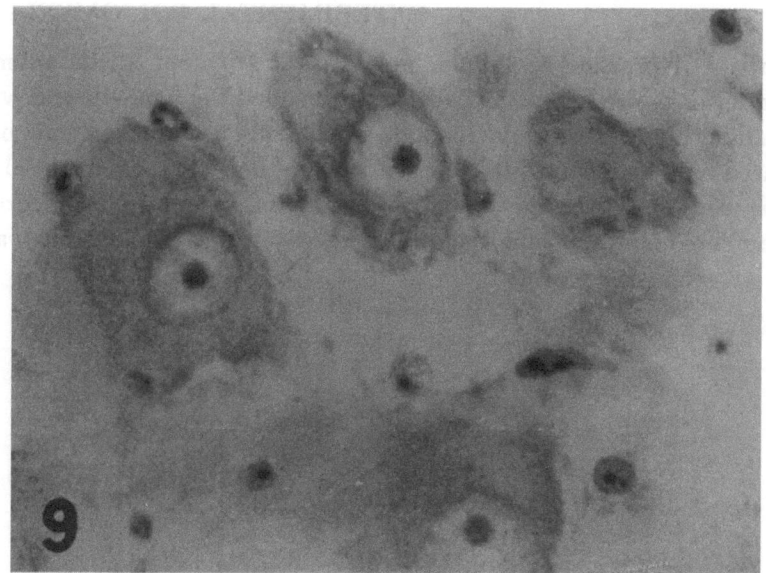

FIGURE 9. POLIOMYELITIS IN THE CORTISONE-TREATED HAMSTER INJECTED INTRAPERITONEALLY
Shows early chromatolysis and some swelling of ganglion cells; thionine ×1100.

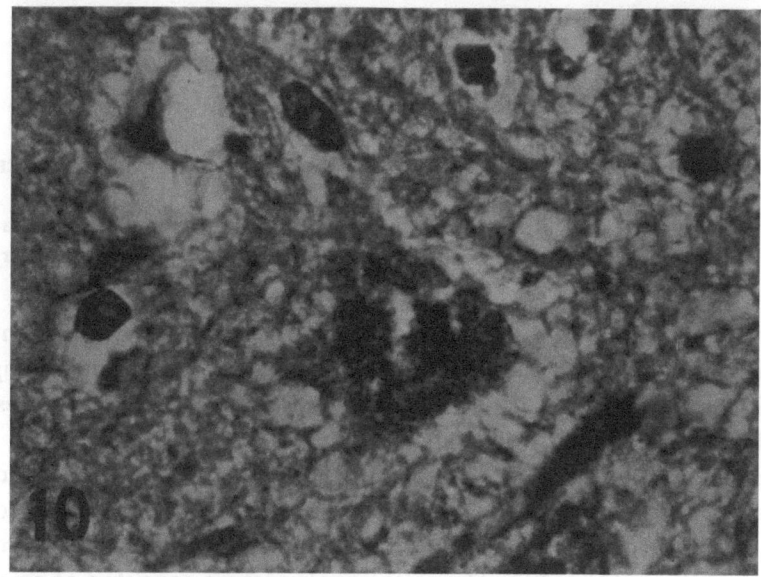

FIGURE 10. POLIOMYELITIS IN THE CORTISONE-TREATED HAMSTER INJECTED INTRAPERITONEALLY
Granular, eosinophilic degeneration of ganglionic cytoplasm and nuclear pyknosis; no inflammatory reaction; H & E ×1100.

ments. A depression of cellular defense was apparent in the anterior horn lesions. The lesions progressively ascended the neuraxis and were usually demonstrable in the medulla when death occurred. In cortisone-treated animals which survived for a longer period of time typical lesions were present as far rostrally as the midbrain and pyriform cortex. These late changes in the brain were mostly patchy and minimal, and

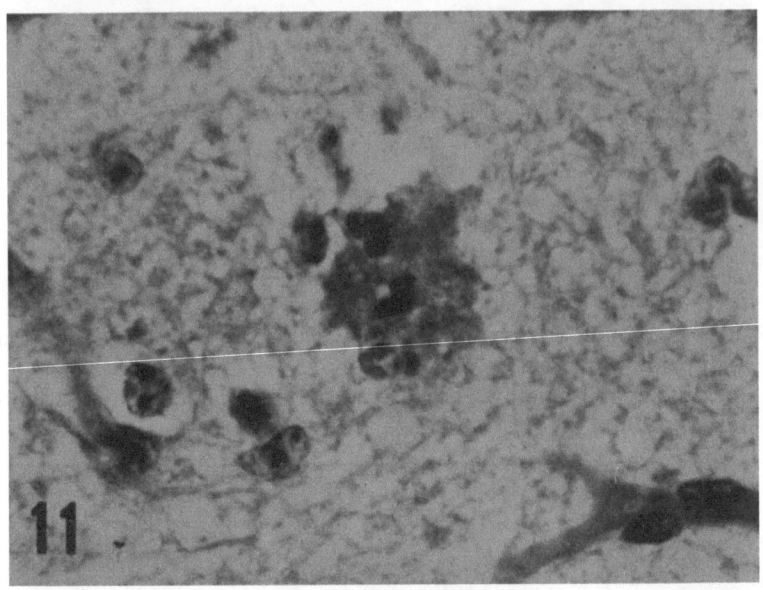

FIGURE 11. POLIOMYELITIS IN THE CORTISONE-TREATED HAMSTER INJECTED INTRAPERITONEALLY
Changes as seen in Fig. 10; a few neutrophile inclusions demonstrable; note quiescent appearance of capillary in right lower corner; H & E ×1100.

never comparable in extent or severity to the lesions evoked by intracerebral injection of the virus. A detailed study of autonomic ganglia within the abdominal cavity failed to incriminate these structures as foci of intermediate involvement.

Histological studies of extraneural tissues demonstrated additional changes found only in MEF_1 inoculated hamsters which received cortisone. The first change was found in the paravertebral and periadrenal adipose tissue (Fig. 13). The microscopic picture consisted of smudginess of the vacuoles and the appearance of minute discrete basophilic bodies lining the inner cell membrane; these granules proceeded rap-

EXPERIMENTAL POLIOMYELITIS

idly to calcification. The interstices, at a later phase, showed the presence of small pleomorphic cells, with moderately abundant basophilic cytoplasm. At a still later stage inflammation supervened, and a foreign-body type of granulomatous reaction was present. Alteration was also noted in skeletal muscle (Fig. 14). The earliest change in this tissue was fading of the cross striations and segmental swelling. In the in-

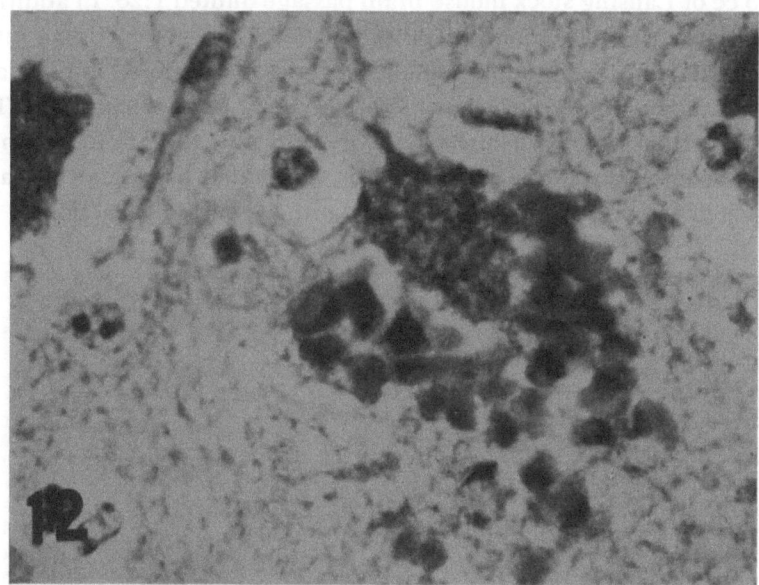

FIGURE 12. POLIOMYELITIS IN THE CORTISONE-TREATED HAMSTER INJECTED INTRAPERITONEALLY
Advanced eosinophilic degeneration of anterior horn ganglion cell; no leukocytic reaction, but hemorrhage into periganglionic space; H & E ×1100.

volved portion of the muscle fiber the swelling sometimes resulted in a fourfold increase in diameter. The myofibrils tended to be maintained for a longer period than were the cross striations, and hyaline-like basophilic masses appeared between these longitudinal structures. Shortly thereafter the fibers fractured, presenting a picture of separated, swollen, and basophilic fragments. This rapidly changed to granular necrosis of the involved sarcoplasm, with an accelerated deposition of calcium. Sarcolemmal cell proliferation around the affected fibers was sometimes present. A dilatory inflammation was obvious at a still later phase. This myositis was localized to the muscles adjacent to the vertebral column.

regardless of whether infection was induced by the intracerebral or the intraperitoneal route (Fig. 13). Both muscle and fat lesions were more severe, however, in the animals infected intraperitoneally. These lesions bear a considerable resemblance to those seen in suckling mice infected with the Coxsackie viruses.

Thirty-seven hamsters were submitted to intraperitoneal inoculation of 0.5 cc of Lansing stock mouse brain passage diluted 1:20. In addition, twenty-seven of these hamsters also received 12 mg of cortisone intramuscularly, divided into four equal doses and administered in two days. The virus was injected at the time of the third dose of cortisone. The Lansing strain is known to be less virulent than the MEF_1 strain. A comparison between the two (in cortisone-treated hamsters) revealed a lower incidence of clinical paralysis and its morbid reflection in the

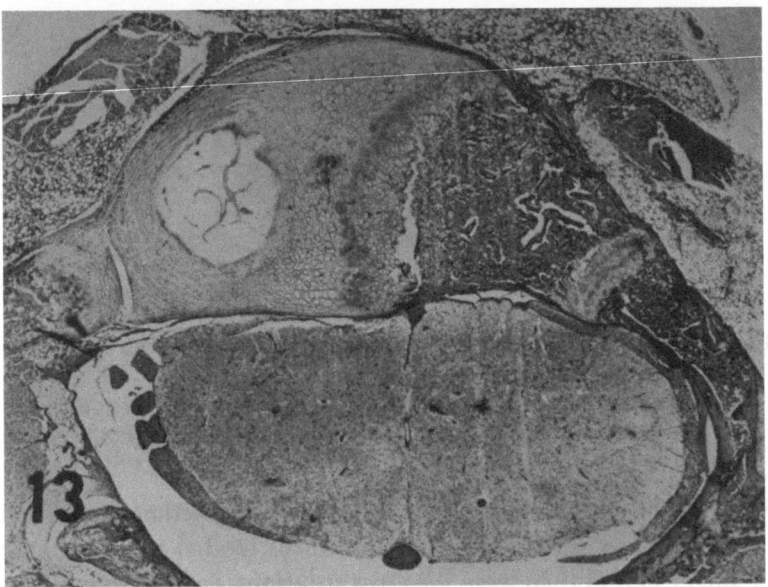

FIGURE 13. LUMBAR SPINAL CORD AND SURROUNDING STRUCTURES IN CORTISONE-TREATED HAMSTER INJECTED INTRAPERITONEALLY WITH MEF_1

Considerable loss of neurons in right anterior horn; some interstitial hemorrhages, but no significant inflammation. Anterior vertebral adipose tissue (upper left and upper right) shows necrosis and minimal inflammatory response; skeletal muscle in same region shows early myositis; H & E ×20.

EXPERIMENTAL POLIOMYELITIS

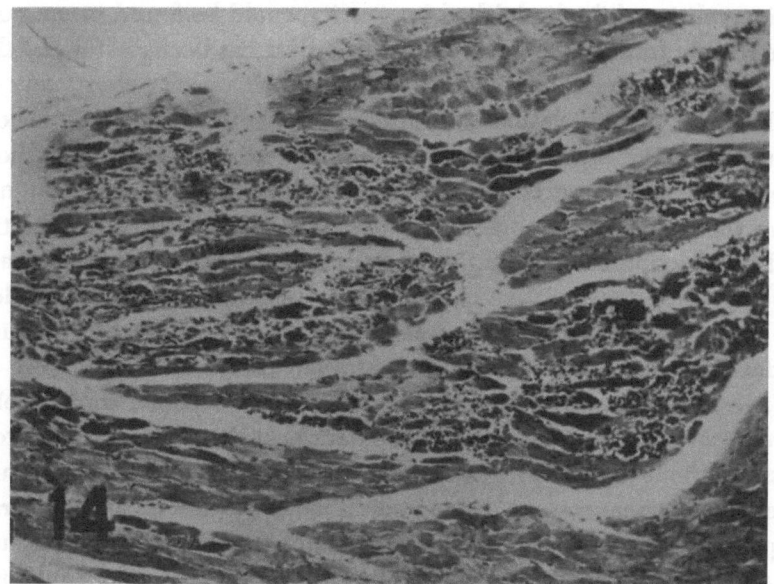

FIGURE 14. PARAVERTEBRAL MUSCLE FROM CORTISONE-TREATED HAMSTER INJECTED INTRAPERITONEALLY WITH MEF_1
Note segmental pattern of involvement. Altered fibers show necrosis, fragmentation, basophilia, and calcification. Some degenerated fibers are surrounded by inflammatory cells. Note resemblance to experimental Coxsackie myositis in the suckling mouse; H & E ×125.

spinal cord in the former group. Statistically significant potentiation, nevertheless, occurred. Approximately 40 percent of the hamsters showed some clinical evidence of paralysis following intraperitoneal inoculation of Lansing virus and intramuscular cortisone. Without supplemental hormones, no paralysis developed. Lytic changes in the anterior horn cells were observed in animals presenting limb paralysis. The myelitis tended to be limited in distribution and intensity. At no time did the damage equal in severity that observed in poliomyelitis caused by the MEF_1 strain. The paravertebral myositis and steatitis described previously was also seen, but again were inconstant and of inappreciable measure. The potentiated disease caused by the MEF_1 strain (intraperitoneally) resulted in paralysis within four days and death usually before the seventh day. Paralysis in cortisone-enhanced Lansing poliomyelitis ensued about the seventh or eighth day, and subsequent mortality was low. In addition, the somatic lesions of Lansing poliomyelitis, while diminished in severity, could be found in musculature remote from the juxtavertebral regions. It has been postulated that the fulminant course of the MEF_1 disease in hamsters aborts any establishment of viral lesions in muscle peripheral to the vertebral column. When the life of the animal is prolonged after inoculation, however, there is a progressive escape of cellular and immune defenses from the influence of cortisone. A dynamic balance of disseminating and constricting forces is achieved in Lansing disease which decreases the degree of degenerative change in any particular locale and widens the distribution of lesions, as compared to MEF_1 poliomyelitis obtained under comparable experimental circumstances.

Investigations pertinent to the action of cortisone upon simian poliomyelitis are in progress. It seems axiomatic that the degree of refractoriness (without cortisone) bears direct correspondence to the magnitude of cortisone enhancement. Intracerebral inoculation of a paralytic strain of poliomyelitis in an adequate concentration into the monkey produces an almost uniformly paralytic disease. Concurrent cortisone results in a decrease of the incubation period and an increase in mortality. The differences achieved are often not striking. However, the potentiation of the disease can be made startlingly demonstrable. Intramuscular inoculation of some strains leads to an extremely low incidence of the disease. Adjuvant cortisone, however, provokes a fulminant disease, tetraplegia, and early death. The full expression of cortisone effects are therefore elicited in the monkey by employing portals of entry which, in the absence of cortisone, would usually fail to eventuate in apparent infection.

Restraint of vascular, inflammatory, and microglial reaction is demonstrable in cortisone-altered monkeys infected with poliomyelitis. Since the simian disease has a longer incubation period and course, as compared to that of the hamster, the inhibition of the above responsive elements is not as prominent in the monkey. However, even in animals sacrificed two weeks after the last injection of cortisone, perivascular cuffing is still meager and the neuronophagia is less extensive. At times the degree of anterior horn damage is so marked as to produce grossly visible cavitary myelomalacia. Topographically, the modified disease is more amplified. After a course of cortisone injections intramuscular inoculation of the Brunhilde strain often results in destruction in all spinal cord levels, devastating damage in the brain stem, bilateral motor cortex changes, and typical lesions of poliomyelitis in the olfactory bulbs. The latter finding creates some misgivings concerning the generally accepted premise of olfactory bulb inviolability following infective routes other than the nasopharyngeal.

The evidence presented points to the vastly important role the host plays in poliomyelitis infection in reference to pathogenesis, the portal of entry, and even the virulence of the virus. The observations reported are by no means limited to poliomyelitis virus. Thus, Kilborne and Horsfall (33) demonstrated an augmented multiplication of influenza A and B and mumps viruses in chick embryos treated with cortisone. They (34) also succeeded in obtaining a fatal Coxsackie disease in cortisone-treated adult mice. The observations of Kilborne and Horsfall were recently confirmed by Findlay and Howard (6). Loosli, Hull, Berlin, and Alexander (35) observed an increase in the mortality rate from air-borne influenza virus in mice receiving ACTH, although there was no alteration in the gross and microscopic findings and in the rate of growth of the virus. On the other hand, the hormone had no effect upon this infection in ferrets (36). It also failed to modify the course of the influenza infection in mice inoculated intranasally, while cortisone treatment increased the mortality rate (37). According to Kalter, Smolin, McElhaney, and Tepperman (38) treatment of mice with ACTH and cortisone caused some depression of multiplication of influenza virus in mice. Cortisone was also reported by Kligman (39) to enhance the vaccinia primary infection and reinfection in guinea pigs. The susceptibility of mice to Japanese B encephalitis was increased in the experiments of Vollmer (40). According to Southam and Babcock (41) cortisone affected adversely the West Nile, Rheus, and Bunyamwera viruses, while ACTH in massive doses also enhanced the West Nile virus. In more recent experiments Findlay and Howard (6) demonstrated the production of extensive liver necrosis following inoculation of Rift Valley fever virus diluted 10^{-6} into cortisone-treated mice. A virus inoculum 10^{-1} was required to produce the same lesion in mice receiving no cortisone. In the experiments of Smith, Murphy, and Mirick (42) the treatment of mice with ACTH did not influence their susceptibility to PVM infection, but slightly enhanced virus multiplication. Cortisone treatment enhanced both the virus infection and the multiplication of virus to a greater degree. Adrenalectomy rendered mice slightly less susceptible to infection and retarded virus growth.

Comparison of the effects of ACTH and cortisone and those of other virus diseases upon poliomyelitis is very difficult at this time in view of the wide divergence of experimental conditions, namely, animal species, time of administration of the hormones, dosage of the hormones, routes used for injection of viruses and so forth. Furthermore, since the hormones have many physiological activities it cannot be assumed that the mechanisms involved in acceleration of infections with viruses widely different from one another are necessarily the same.

REFERENCES

This bibliography embodies papers which were reported before the date of the Symposium.

1. Curley, F. J., and W. L. Aycock, The effect of stilbestrol on resistance to experimental poliomyelitis, *Endocrinology*, 1946, 39:414.
2. Venning, E. H., Adrenal function in pregnancy, *Endocrinology*, 1946, 39:203.
3. Shwartzman, G., Enhancing effect of cortisone upon poliomyelitis infection (strain MEF_1) in hamsters and mice, *Proc. Soc. Exp. Biol. & Med.*, 1950, 75:835.
4. Shwartzman, G., and A. Fisher, Alteration of experimental poliomyelitis infection in the Syrian hamster with the aid of cortisone, *J. Exp. Med.*, 1952, 95:347.
5. Sabin, A. B., Genetic, hormonal and age factors in natural resistance to certain viruses, *Ann. N.Y. Acad. Sci.*, 1952, 54:936.
6. Findlay, G. M., and E. M. Howard, The effects of cortisone and adrenocorticotropic hormone on poliomyelitis and on other virus infections, *J. Pharm. Lond.*, 1952, 4:37.
7. Levinson, S. O., A. Milzer, and P. Lewin, Effect of fatigue, chilling and mechanical trauma on resistance to experimental poliomyelitis, *Am. J. Hyg.*, 1945, 42:204.
8. Russel, W. R., Poliomyelitis. The pre-paralytic stage, and the effect of physical activity on the severity of paralysis, *Brit. Med. J.*, 1947, 2:1023.
9. Horstmann, D. M., Acute poliomyelitis; relation of physical activity at the time of onset to the course of the infection, *J.A.M.A.*, 1950, 142:236.
10. Aycock, W. L., Tonsillectomy and poliomyelitis; I: Epidemiologic considerations, *Medicine*, 1942, 21:65.
11. Francis, T., Jr., C. E. Krill, J. A. Toomey, and W. N. Mack, Poliomyelitis following tonsillectomy in five members of a family; an epidemiologic study, *J.A.M.A.*, 1942, 119:1392.
12. Magnus, H. von, and J. L. Melnick, Tonsillectomy in experimental poliomyelitis, *Am. J. Hyg.*, 1948, 48:113.
13. Faber, H. K., McNaught, R. C., R. J. Silverberg, and L. Dong, Experi-

mental production of post-tonsillectomy bulbar poliomyelitis, *Proc. Soc. Exp. Biol. & Med.*, 1951, 77:532.
14. Harrington, A. B., Paralytic poliomyelitis following injury, *Lancet*, 1951, 260:987.
15. McGoogan, L. S., Acute anterior poliomyelitis, complicating pregnancy, *Am. J. Obst. & Gynec.*, 1932, 24:215.
16. Aycock, W. L., The frequency of poliomyelitis in pregnancy, *New England J. Med.*, 1941, 225:405.
17. Aycock, W. L., Acute poliomyelitis in pregnancy; its occurence according to the month of pregnancy and sex of fetus, *New England J. Med.*, 1946, 235:160.
18. Byrd, C. L., Jr., The influence of infection with Lansing strain poliomyelitis virus on pregnant mice, *J. Neuropath. & Exp. Neurol.*, 1950, 9:202.
19. Knox, L., Influence of pregnancy in mice on the course of infection with murine poliomyelitis virus, *Proc. Soc. Exp. Biol. & Med.*, 1950, 73:520.
20. Geffen, D. B., The incidence of paralysis occurring in London children within four weeks after immunization, *Med. Off.*, Lond., 1950, 83:137.
21. Hill, A. B., and J. Knowelden, Inoculation and poliomyelitis; a statistical investigation in England and Wales in 1949, *Brit. Med. J.*, 1950, 2:1.
22. McCloskey, B. P., The relation of prophylactic inoculations to the onset of poliomyelitis, *Lancet*, 1950, 258:659.
23. Martin, J. K., Local paralysis in children after injections, *Arch. Dis. Childhood*, 1950, 25:1.
24. Anderson, G. W., and A. E. Skaar, Poliomyelitis occurring after antigen injections, *Bull. Univ. Minn. Hosp. & Minn. Med. Found.*, 1951, 22:359.
25. Goerke, L. S., The precipitation of clinical poliomyelitis by injections, *Calif. J. Med.*, 1951, 74:383.
26. Findlay, G. M., and E. M. Howard, Non-specific shock in experimental poliomyelitis, *J. Path. & Bact.*, 1950, 62:371.
27. Milzer, A., M. A. Weiss, and K. Vanderboom, Effect of pertussis, diphtheria toxoid and salmonella immunization on experimental poliomyelitis, *Proc. Soc. Exp. Biol. & Med.*, 1951, 77:485.
28. Coriell, L. L., A. C. Siegel, C. D. Cook, L. Murphy, and J. Stokes, Jr., Use of pituitary adrenocorticotrophic hormone (ACTH) in poliomyelitis, *J.A.M.A.*, 1950, 142:1279.
29. Ainslie, J. D., T. Francis, Jr., and G. C. Brown, ACTH in experimental poliomyelitis in monkeys and mice, *J. Lab. & Clin. Med.*, 1951, 38:344.
30. Foster, C., M. M. Sigel, W. Henle, and J. Stokes, Jr., The influence of ACTH on the resistance of monkeys to the Yale SK strain of poliomyelitis virus, *J. Lab. & Clin. Med.*, 1951, 38:359.
31. Bodian, D., Pathogenesis of poliomyelitis in normal and passively immunized primates after virus feeding, *Fed. Proc.*, 1952, 11:462.
32. Horstmann, D. M., Poliomyelitis virus in the blood of orally infected monkeys and chimpanzees, *Fed. Proc.*, 1952, 11:471.

33. Kilborne, E. D., and F. L. Horsfall, Jr., Increased virus in eggs injected with cortisone, *Proc. Soc. Exp. Biol. & Med.*, 1951, 76:116.
34. Kilborne, E. D., and F. L. Horsfall, Jr., Lethal infection with Coxsackie virus of adult mice given cortisone, *Proc. Soc. Exp. Biol. & Med.*, 1951, 77:135.
35. Loosli, C. G., R. B. Hull, B. S. Berlin, and E. R. Alexander, The influence of ACTH on the course of experimental influenza type A virus, *J. Lab. & Clin. Med.*, 1951, 37:464.
36. Hull, R. B., and C. G. Loosli, Adrenocorticotrophic hormone (ACTH) in the treatment of experimental air-borne influenza virus type A infection in the ferret, *J. Lab. & Clin. Med.*, 1951, 37:603.
37. Kass, E. H., S. H. Ingbar, M. M. Lundgren, and M. Finland, The effect of ACTH and cortisone on pneumococcal and influenza viral infections in the white mouse, *J. Lab. & Clin. Med.*, 1951, 37:780.
38. Kalter, S. S., H. J. Smolin, J. M. McElhaney, and J. Tepperman, Endocrines and their relation to influenza virus infection, *J. Exp. Med.*, 1951, 93:529.
39. Kligman, A. M., G. D. Baldridge, G. Rebell, and D. M. Pillsbury, The effect of cortisone on the pathologic responses of guinea pigs infected cutaneously with fungi, viruses, and bacteria, *J. Lab. & Clin. Med.*, 1951, 37:615.
40. Vollmer, E. P., and H. S. Hurlbut, Ineffectiveness of cortisone therapy in mice infected with Japanese B encephalitis and the adverse effect of high doses, *J. Inf. Dis.*, 1951, 89:103.
41. Southam, C. M., and V. I. Babcock, Effect of cortisone, related hormones, and adrenalectomy on susceptibility of mice to virus infections, *Proc. Soc. Exp. Biol. & Med.*, 1951, 78:105.
42. Smith, J. M., J. S. Murphy, and G. S. Mirick, Effect of adrenal hormones on infection of mice with pneumonia virus of mice (PVM), *Proc. Soc. Exp. Biol. & Med.*, 1951, 78:505.

SYMPOSIA OF

THE SECTION ON MICROBIOLOGY

THE NEW YORK ACADEMY OF MEDICINE

1. Diagnosis of Viral and Rickettsial Infections
   Edited by Frank L. Horsfall, Jr.

2. Evaluation of Chemotherapeutic Agents
   Edited by Colin M. MacLeod

3. The Pathogenesis and Pathology of Viral Diseases
   Edited by John G. Kidd

4. Parasitic Infections in Man
   Edited by Harry Most

5. The Nature and Significance of the Antibody Response
   Edited by A. M. Pappenheimer, Jr.

6. The Effect of ACTH and Cortisone upon Infection and Resistance
   Edited by Gregory Shwartzman

Bei Fragen zur Produktsicherheit wenden Sie sich bitte an:
If you have any questions regarding product safety,
please contact:

Walter de Gruyter GmbH
Genthiner Straße 13
10785 Berlin
productsafety@degruyterbrill.com